Hair Network

Confessions From A Hair Salon

LUCILLE FORDIN

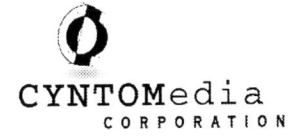

CYNTOMedia CORPORATION

Pittsburgh, PA

CeShore

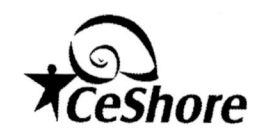

ISBN 1-58501-086-3

Trade Paperback
© Copyright 2004 Lucille Fordin
All rights reserved
First Printing—2004
Library of Congress #2004106637

Request for information should be addressed to:

SterlingHouse Publisher, Inc.
7436 Washington Avenue
Pittsburgh, PA 15218
www.sterlinghousepublisher.com

CeShore is an imprint of SterlingHouse Publisher, Inc.

SterlingHouse Publisher, Inc. is a company
of the CyntoMedia Corporation

Art Director: Matthew J. Lorenz
Cover Design: Matthew J. Lorenz - SterlingHouse Publisher
Typesetting & Layout Design: N. J. McBeth
Illustration/Cover Art: Matthew J. Lorenz

All rights reserved. No part of this publication may be reproduced, stored in a retrieval system, or transmitted in any form or by any means—electronic, mechanical, photocopy, recording or any other, except for brief quotations in printed reviews—without prior permission of the publisher.

Printed in the United States of America

Dedication

I dedicate this book to my family, especially my two nephews whom I love to death, and to everyone else who said I was too stupid to make anything out of my life. Guess what? The joke's on you.

To Betty,
My life is now in your hands.
Love
Lucy

Table of Contents

1. Welcome To The World of Hair Network
2. No Underwear, But Still He Covered His Ass
3. The Beauty Contestant And The Evil Eye
4. Gina, Tina And Jekyll And Hyde
5. All My Children
6. Condo Tragedies
7. A Stiff Dick Has No Conscience
8. Having Your Cake And Wearing It Too
9. One Of The Best Kept Secrets I Ever Heard – From A $500 Pee To A Law Degree
10. Big Banana's Foster
11. Hot Fudge For A Hot Potato
12. Have The Lizards And Frogs Stood Up And Applauded You Yet?
13. Tarzan Wants To Pump You Up
14. I Want My Two Hundred Bucks Back
15. Jill, The Blonde, And The Pill
16. Who Do You Trust?
17. Like A Bunch Of Dirty Old School Boys
18. My Sweet Karate Blocks
19. He Loves Me Like My Mother Loved Me
20. You're Italian, You Must Know Someone
21. Florida Grandmas Are Not Baking Bread Or Making Meatballs
22. Everyone Has Someone Somewhere

23. Just One Of The Girls And The Disease To Please
24. What Was That Noise I Heard Larry?
25. Now Who Would Buy Somebody A Car On A Maybe?
26. Sometimes People Make Mistakes – Otherwise Known As The Beth Principle
27. Like An Angel With A Smile On Her Face
28. Keep The Tranquilizers Coming Girls!
29. I've Never Seen Lips As Big As My Feet Before
30. I'm Next
31. You Don't Have To Be A Genius

Gossip! Gossip! Gossip! Who doesn't love gossip? This book is a selection of *some* of the juicy stories I've been told in my hair salon over the years by everyday people just like you and me. These stories are all true. You may or may not agree with some of my beliefs as they unfold throughout the book. From the good to the bad, and let's not forget the ugly! OOPS, have I slipped already?

As you'll see, one of my beliefs is that women are the hidden power of the world. I'll show you how real people can live through being raped, abused, mentally tortured, and then miraculously turn their lives around and actually survive the streets. I'm going to tell you stories about children, teenagers, and adults, about men and women, about the rich and the poor. The way I see it, life is all about winners, losers, and yes, wannabes.

My life has been motivated by a powerful American fear: The fear of being poor. Another belief I have is that love and laughter conquer all. I'm sure you've experienced how good it feels to, on occasion, just throw your head back and laugh hysterically. I think it's very healthy. Finally, I know if I can make it in this life, so can you. So just stop complaining and do it! This is my story....

Chapter One:
Welcome To The World of Hair Network

I'm ready now to welcome you into the world of Hair Network. Let's see if you can relate to any or all of these stories. You know, a hairdresser is trusted in the same way that you would trust your doctor. People tell us their most private and personal feelings about everything from their sex life to their aches and pains. I'm going to tell you some stories I remember as though they just happened yesterday.

Hair Network is a happy, fun, professional beauty salon. I make holidays spectacular by having a full buffet all week. At Christmas, there are gifts at the door for every client, presents under the tree for the children, and a drawing for a free hair blow and manicure by each stylist and manicurist, just to show clients my appreciation. I believe every client should be treated with respect. Most of our clients are retired. Teenagers, judges and models, lawyers, gamblers, policewomen, entertainers, strippers, secretaries, stockbrokers, travel agents… you name it, they come into my salon. They come from every state, country, and island on this planet. I have men and women from all walks of life, some with a lot of money, some without, some with class, and some without. To me, people are very important and need special attention, especially when they come to a beauty salon. I must pay close attention to their lifestyles, the way they dress, talk, walk, and act. It gives me an idea of how to do their hair to make them happy. I make sure they leave the salon feeling beautiful. A hairdresser has to be a magician sometimes and a good psychologist most of the time.

I feel Mother's Day, Halloween, Christmas, and Hanukkah are good times to celebrate in the salon. My Hair Network parties are my special way of showing my appreciation to my employees and to all the clients.

Lucille Fordin

On Mother's Day, I have a complete buffet the entire week. Mothers are special to me, as they are to everyone else. To me, mothers are the real strength of this world.

Halloween is a blast! I decorate the entire salon. Employees come to work dressed in costumes, and as I've mentioned, beauticians are quite the artists, so you should see some of their elaborate, wild and wacky, sometimes quite convincing, costumes. Each employee brings a favorite dish that they prepare themselves. We have a party that people talk about for three months.

When you come into the salon, you'll find twenty-five platters of food from all over the world, plus desserts galore, which I make myself.

My employees are from all over the world: Italy, Cuba, Israel, France, Russia, Bahamas, United States and Germany. Some speak many languages. I only speak English, and I enjoy learning about their families and how different their lives were before coming to the United States. I can't imagine waiting in lines for bread in Russia and not being able to express an opinion on politics. One hairdresser was living barefoot in Cuba with nine family members until she was eighteen and came to the United States. People who come from Israel are very aggressive and stick together like glue. I understand being in the Army for two years can change anyone; it's a real learning experience. Hair Network is a fine international hair salon for an international state.

At Christmas time, I go crazy. I decorate the mirrors, the ceiling, the windows... you name it, I decorate it. I put up a Christmas tree and I have a complete Hanukkah section for our Jewish clientele. The buffet goes on all week.

Christmas at Hair Network starts with a gala dinner for the employees and their spouses or dates. The evening out makes us all feel good. We get to dance, and after a few drinks, conga lines are circling the lounge at the Country Club.

One year, I was passing out bonuses to my staff and grab bags were being exchanged. Everyone was opening presents. I was being kissed and thanked for a great year when I was presented with the most beautiful sculpture from Italy; it was a gift from all of the employees.

Three days later the party began in the salon. Tuesday through Saturday there was a complete buffet from 8am to 6pm. All the clients are welcome to eat. I prepared everything, except for a few items. The buffet consisted of lasagna, meatballs, sausage, three different pasta salads, coleslaw, sandwiches, chopped liver, chicken salad, and bagels, naturally. There are plenty of garnishes, cakes, candies, cookies, Danishes, muffins, and fudge balls.

Not too many salons in this world show this much appreciation to their clients for their patronage. Women and men spend a lot of time and money on their hair. I love to thank them in my own way.

For five weeks, clients put their names in a Christmas box. Fifteen gift bags with lovely presents and ten facials are given to the twenty-five lucky winners, along with a gift at the door.

I see now after twenty years in business why bosses lose their mind. Pressure, big time. I have always wanted to believe if I'm good to everyone, then they'll be good to me. Wrong again. How naïve could I be?

When you're dealing with the general public, not to mention very artistic employees who think they do a better job than you, trust me, it's not easy. Adults in general think they know it all. I should have known my life would never be easy. But the way I look at it, my life can be as hard or as easy as I want it to be. I love people. I respect my employees, and I must say I'm not a bad boss. I have parties all the time, and I'm sure to make birthdays very special. We have a lot of fun at Hair Network.

I try hard to keep the employees, along with the clients, in an upbeat mood. I make jokes out of situations that cause an employee to flip. If a woman doesn't like one of my staff's work, I try to place her with another hairdresser or manicurist. This causes me problems with my employees. Employees only look at what their paycheck is and not at the overall good of the salon. I have signs up that say, "Feel free to switch operators, not salons."

It's a very uncomfortable situation when someone has to switch. Clients are uncomfortable and employees feel they're not good enough. So I watch the client and employee for a few weeks until the client is set with another operator. One person's loss is another's gain, and I protect the salon by keeping the client happy.

If an employee has a personal problem or doctor's appointment, etc. and has to leave during the day for an hour or two, I let her go as long as she moves her clients to another time. I let everyone bring their families

Lucille Fordin

in at no charge, and if an employee needs to do a favor for someone, I let her charge less or not at all. I trust my employees' judgement.

I learned what I, as an employee, didn't like from prior bosses. One boss threw brushes across the room every time a client didn't like her hair. One day I got hit with one of the brushes, and that was the end of that job.

Another boss was sleeping with all the clients. Nero was a gorgeous Greek guy. I'll never forget him, even though this was back in my Pittsburgh days. He said to me, "If you don't fuck me you won't be here long." Naturally I thought he was joking. He was constantly putting his hands on me and everyone else. The women threw themselves at him. At least three times a day women would call the salon and say they were sick, "Could Nero make a house call?" Nero was billing a hundred dollars an hour in 1970. I couldn't understand why these women would take a chance of getting a disease or destroying their marriages over a hairdresser. I mean, everyone knew what he was doing.

I was able to put him off for six months until one night when I had to work late. I really needed the job. My father was out of work, and being the oldest child, I always felt the need to be the caretaker.

I had just finished my last client when Nero said, "I need to speak to you." My heart was pounding and I was scared to death. I thought he was going to fire me. I never would have dreamt what was about to happen.

Nero said to me, "Lucy, you're young and you have a lot to learn. I won't let you work here unless you fuck me."

I was terrified, and said to him, "What do you mean, I'm not good enough? You know I'm better than you and I'm not sleeping with all the clients. If you fire me, I'll tell everyone you gave me a sex ultimatum and you'll really be in a lot of trouble."

Just then he grabbed me by my arms and pulled me to his body. "You stupid kid," he said. "Everyone wants my body. I want you now." Nero pushed his lips against mine and shoved his tongue down my throat.

"I'm hot for you, baby, get your clothes off now." I wasn't scared anymore. I was mad, and knew I had to think fast and outsmart him.

I smiled at him and said, "Okay Nero, you get undressed. You're in for the ride of your life."

As Nero was taking off his pants, the biggest penis I had ever seen in my life came flying out and stood at attention. I didn't know whether to salute it or grab my scissors and cut it off. As Nero bent down to take his leg out of his pants, I decided to run as fast as I could out the door.

The next day I called in sick and decided to go over to my mother's place to tell her what happened. She went crazy.

"Lucy, don't ever tell your father because he'll end up in jail. He'll shoot first and ask questions later. Now I on the other hand will be nice and just cut his dick off." Mom always made me laugh no matter how bad the situation was. I was only 20 years old and had a lot to learn.

Mom said, "Get in the car now. We're going over there. I'll scare that son of a bitch so bad he'll never get a hard-on again. Lucy, when a woman says no, it means no. No job is worth your dignity."

As we pulled up to the shop, there were police everywhere. The hairdressers and clients were being questioned. Nero was being taken away in an ambulance. We could see blood everywhere. We ran up to Amy the receptionist and I asked what happened.

Amy said there had been a terrible fight in the salon and Nero had been hurt. She said that at ten o'clock Mrs. Solomon had called and asked if Nero could make a house call. "Naturally he said yes. 'I'll be there at one o'clock.' Nero got back to the salon at two-thirty. Apparently Mr. Solomon came home early and caught them together. Nero denied everything and left. At three o'clock Mr. Solomon came in the door like a maniac. He grabbed Nero and just beat the living shit out of him. Then he broke his arm."

My mom said, "Oh shit, now I can't cut his dick off." Nero was out of commission for a long time. He lost his business because all of his hairdressers moved to another salon and their clients followed.

My first year in business was a real hum-dinger! Pepe's hair salon was my only competition. His salon had been in business for five years and he was very busy. There were nine little salons in the area.

One day a short Italian man came through the front door of the salon like gangbusters. He was speaking loudly and was very aggressive when he approached my receptionist. "Get the owner up here now," he said.

Lucille Fordin

The clients and employees got scared and there was dead silence for a moment. Everyone's head turned toward the front of the shop, including mine.

I was doing a haircut when all of a sudden my hand slipped. I was startled from the commotion and my scissors cut my client's necklace off her neck. The necklace fell into her lap. Her eyes opened wide and her mouth dropped open. She was in shock and so was I. I immediately started to apologize and told her I would pay to fix it. I knew a $200 gold chain had just cost me $1,000, so I was really pissed off.

I dropped everything and started running to the front desk. It looked like I was in a marathon. I heard a client say, "Stay calm, everyone. That shrimp is going to be dead meat once Lucy gets up there. I bet $5 on Lucy." Everyone started pulling money out, betting on the shrimp or Lucy.

I was eye to eye with him. He had brown eyes, dark skin, black hair and was wearing tight black leather pants and a black silk shirt. He looked like Mafia.

I said to him, "Sir, lower your voice and tell me what your problem is. My name is Lucy. I own this salon. And your name is…?"

He said, "Pepe. I own Pepe's salon. I'm sick of my clients leaving me and coming to this stupid salon. Women shouldn't be in business. You're all stupid and should be home making babies, especially a bimbo like you. If you think I'll let you hurt my business, you're making a big mistake. I'll run you out of town first, bimbo."

I pointed to the door and screamed back, "Pepe, we'll see about that. Now get out of my shop and don't let the door hit you in the ass."

Pepe stormed out the door while saying, "I'm not done with you yet, bitch."

Everyone in the salon started applauding and I bowed and said, "Let the games begin."

Chapter Two:
No Underwear, But Still He Covered His Ass

It's time to put some spice in your life! Maybe someone in your family has experimented in ways you wouldn't have believed 'til you heard about it from the horse's mouth. You just never know what some people will do for a little bit of fun and excitement.

It was February 14th, Valentine's Day, and a glorious day in Miami. The sun was reflecting off the trees while they danced from left to right as the breeze blew from the ocean. I was in my car on my way to the salon, wondering what was in store for me that day. Was it going to be a good day or a bad day? All of a sudden the big black Lincoln Continental in front of me stopped dead in the street and my car crashed into its fender. Well, I guess that answered what kind of day I was going to have.

As soon as I realized I was okay, I looked up and noticed that the man in the Lincoln in front of me wasn't moving. I quickly grabbed my cell phone and dialed 911, thinking he was dead. I frantically jumped out of the car to see if I could help him. I started knocking on the window, screaming, "Are you okay? Unlock the door." All of a sudden a cute blonde around thirty years old popped up her head and there was semen all over her chin. The man turned his head toward me and said, "It was worth wrecking my car for that. What a great Valentine's Day present I just got. I just had the best orgasm of my life!"

My mouth dropped open in shock when I noticed that the cute little blonde was Yolanda, a client from the salon.

"Yolanda, is that you underneath all that stuff on your face? I called 911. I thought this gentleman had a heart attack and was dead."

Just then, Best-Orgasm-In-My-Life looked up at me and said with a blissful smile, "What a way to go! Don't worry about your car. Put your insurance card away. I'll pay for everything. Yolanda, do you know this gal?"

"Yes, it's Lucy. She owns the salon I go to. Lucy, let me introduce you to my boyfriend, Paul."

"Yolanda, we have to get out of here fast; there's something I never told you," Paul said.

"Paul, I'm sure it can wait. Are you sure you aren't hurt? There's blood on your penis."

"Yolanda, you vampire, you bit me."

I felt like I was in a bad movie. I was very nervous and I blurted out, "Hey, guys, I called 911. An ambulance is on the way."

Paul had a look of panic on his face and said, "Yolanda, listen to me. You have to get out of here . . . I'm married."

"Married!" Yolanda screamed. "You son of a bitch! You men are all the same! I thought you loved me. I wish I had bitten your dick off!"

"Paul," I asked, "do I know you? You look very familiar to me. Have you ever been in my salon?"

"What's the name of your salon?"

"Hair Network," I replied. When I realized that he was Mr. Artfield, a client's husband, I called him on it. Paul looked like he'd just seen a ghost . . . his own.

"Mr. Artfield, it can't possibly be you. Your wife will die if she finds out about this. How are you going to explain the teeth marks on that soon-to-be-dead dick of yours? Well, I guess you can say your zipper bit you. I have a client who's a nurse and she tells me at least 50 guys a year come into the emergency room, wearing no underwear, with their penis stuck in their zipper." Paul and Yolanda burst out laughing at this until tears came into their eyes.

"Yolanda, please get out of the car fast before the ambulance arrives."

"Listen to him, Yolanda. I'll take you home. Paul's wife is a wonderful woman; she doesn't deserve this kind of pain."

Yolanda sobbed as she said, "No! He deserves to get caught. He said he would marry me."

"Yolanda, please listen to Lucy. We'll work everything out later. I'll get a divorce, I promise. I love you. Please don't let my family find out this way."

"Please, Yolanda, come with me," I said. "I hear the ambulance coming. Do it for Paul before the police get here. You don't want this to hit the newspapers. It would be embarrassing for you."

She hesitated at first but finally said, "Okay. I'm doing this for me and you, Lucy, not for him."

As I drove away, I couldn't help thinking about Mrs. Artfield's reaction to finding out that her husband wrecked the Linclon while getting a blowjob.

The next month would prove to be very stressful because of this situation, especially since Yolanda and Mrs. Artfield were both regular clients in the salon.

Yolanda cried all the way home. She said over and over again, "I love him. I hate him. I'll kill him if he doesn't marry me. And then I'll kill myself."

"Yolanda, you're only thirty-two and there's plenty of good men out there. Don't give up yet," I said. "Women can be bigger whores than men sometimes. You can't be blamed. In my opinion, men somehow forget to mention one important detail, mind you the most important one, that they're married. To them it's a little white lie. Yolanda, my mother, who was a smart woman, always told me to remember this: 'A stiff dick has no conscience.' It's like men are collecting trophies. Climax, climax, climax. Score, score, score. Another trophy! Hooray! Yolanda, you must realize most men never leave their wives because they don't want to endanger the stability of family life, not to mention the settlement they'd have to pay."

"Lucy, Paul loves me. He'll leave his wife, you'll see. Please tell me what Paul's wife looks like. Is she pretty? I hope she's fat and ugly. Please tell me."

"Yolanda, what good would it do to know what she looks like? It's not her fault, you know, it's his. Anyway, I don't want to see you hurt any more than you are right now."

"Lucy, I really love Paul. I've been seeing him for a whole year and I know his businesses are all over the world. I see him at least four nights a week. He bought me a new car and a condo. I feel so stupid telling you all this. He set me up in a little business. He's only fifty-eight years old and he works very hard . . . Please Lucy, tell me what she looks like."

Lucille Fordin

"Yolanda, I've known Cindy for seven years now. The whole family comes into the salon. Cindy happens to be a quiet, sweet, lovely woman who lives only for her husband and their kids. She's thin and blonde, and also very rich."

"Lucy, please point her out to me at the salon."

"Absolutely not, Yolanda. I've known you for three years and I've grown very fond of you. But if I'm right, Paul will never tell his wife. Paul has too much to lose and he loves money. Cindy's father owned the business and turned it over to Paul and Cindy. In divorce or death, Cindy gets everything."

"Lucy, how do you know all of this for sure?"

"Yolanda, it's a small world we live in, and people never stop talking about other people. I can't help myself from listening to all the stories. I'm not telling you anything that everyone doesn't already know. Now, about Paul and Cindy's family, I'm sure if you ask around, you'll hear the same gossip I just told you. And I can't afford any trouble at the salon. I'm your friend, but I also have a business to run."

"Easy for you to say, Lucy. Paul got his Valentine's Day present from me in the car and now I'm left high and dry. I'm screwed out of a present."

I couldn't believe this girl was worried about a present while her life had just been turned upside down.

A few days later while Renaldo was doing Yolanda's hair, I heard her ask Renaldo when Cindy came in to get her hair done. She never stopped asking until she found out.

Two weeks later Yolanda was at the salon and I noticed Cindy was due to arrive for her hair appointment any minute. I predicted this would eventually happen. It was inevitable. I decided to get involved by calling Cindy and telling her a fib, that Renaldo was running late and not to come until two hours later. Yolanda finished her manicure and was still hanging around a long time when I walked up to her and said, "Yolanda, if you're waiting for Cindy to come in, you're wasting your time. She cancelled her appointment." Another fib. "You promised me you wouldn't cause any trouble in the salon."

"Lucy, how did you find out I was waiting for her?"

"It's obvious, and besides, my receptionist Rosie is my best friend. She told me you kept asking everyone, 'when does Cindy come in?' By the way, how's Paul's penis?"

"I don't know, Lucy, he went on a business trip."

"I wonder how he explained the teeth marks. I've already received a generous check from Paul to get my car repaired. I can see why you're so in love with him. He's very charming and handsome."

A week later Paul came back from his trip and told Yolanda he was leaving his wife and would marry her. Paul bought Yolanda a new Jaguar and a beautiful four-carat engagement ring. She was happier than I had ever seen her.

Later in the week Cindy came into the salon. While Renaldo was doing her hair, all I could hear was Cindy and Renaldo laughing hysterically.

I couldn't stand it any longer so I flew over to Renaldo's chair to see what was going on. "Cindy, now that the whole shop is laughing, you have to tell me what's so funny. I could use a good laugh."

"Lucy, Paul had a car accident." I broke out into a sweat and got very nervous and said to myself, I'm dead meat now, but why the laughing? I said to Cindy, "That doesn't sound so funny to me. Is Paul okay?" Cindy and Renaldo burst out laughing all over again. I looked at the two of them very puzzled and said, "You two are crazy."

Then Cindy jumped in and said, "Lucy, you don't understand. Paul was in the car rushing to a meeting when he noticed his zipper was opened. When he went to zip his pants, his penis got stuck in his zipper and he slammed on his brakes. The car hit a telephone pole and off he went into the ambulance to get his penis freed from his zipper."

Now we were all laughing so hard we were crying. I was relieved, but still felt bad for lying.

"They told Paul at the hospital that it's very dangerous for a man not to wear underwear and that penises getting stuck in zippers is a very common problem. I've gotten a lot of rest this week, if you know what I mean. The poor thing is all bruised up and very sore. No sex for a couple of weeks, so Paul decided to take me to Europe next month. Look what it takes to get him to go on vacation. He works so hard."

Lucille Fordin

All of a sudden a woman in rollers in the next chair hollered out, "What happened to his underwear, dear? Are you just a dummy? Who was he parking with?"

I could have killed that customer. Cindy was beside herself. Being the lady that she is, she answered very innocently, "Paul has a bad stomach. He couldn't make it to the bathroom on time, so he threw his underwear in the garbage and kept on going to the office."

It took a couple of weeks until Yolanda heard this story. By then Paul and Cindy were in Europe. Paul naturally told Yolanda he was going on a business trip alone. Yolanda was having her nails done when she heared another woman say, "How lucky Cindy is to have such a wonderful man. He gets his dick stuck in his zipper and then takes her to Europe because he can't have sex with her for a couple of weeks. I bet they're having fun making up for lost time."

I saw the pain on Yolanda's face as she paid her bill and left without saying a word. Later that evening I received a phone call from Yolanda. She was very drunk and out of her mind. I could barely understand her. Her words were slurred. "Are you doing drugs?" I asked her.

"I hate that mother fucker," she blurted out. "I'll kill his wife, then his kids."

"Yolanda, stop! Calm down."

"I have a gun. I'm going to kill myself."

"No, Yolanda, let me get you some help." She kept screaming and crying. "No one can help me. I don't want to live. I'll kill Paul and then I'll kill myself."

Then there was dead silence. "Yolanda, are you there? Speak to me. Are you all right? Talk to me." There was no reply. I kept thinking, Please be alive. I hung up and called 911. I jumped in the car and drove to Yolanda's condo, almost killing myself as I ran a red light. The ambulance arrived at the same time I did. We were pounding on the door when a neighbor came out and said, "I have a key."

As we opened the door and ran in, it looked like a war zone. The condo was destroyed. Yolanda was lying half on the couch and half on the floor. We didn't know if she had passed out or if she were dead. Her hair was a mess and her makeup was smeared all over her face. Broken lamps and dishes lay all over the floor. Empty liquor bottles, cocaine and sleeping pills were on the coffee table. My feet were frozen to the floor.

The next thing I heard was one of the emergency guys saying, "I've lost her pulse." They worked on her and got her breathing again and quickly rushed her to the hospital. It was a close call, but she made it. The empty bottles of Scotch, drugs and sleeping pills she took almost killed her. She later said a friend gave her the pills, but she never said where the other drugs came from.

Yolanda was in bad shape for a week and definitely needed psychiatric care. She kept repeating, "I'm in love with Paul. How could he lie to me and then take his wife to Europe?"

A week later I received a beautiful bouquet of flowers with a thank you note for saving Yolanda's life and going every day to the hospital. Yolanda was doing well and said she never wanted to see Paul again.

A week later Paul returned to the States, dropped his wife off at home, and naturally went straight to Yolanda's. As he unlocked the door with his key, he sensed something was wrong and a chill ran through his body. Paul started screaming, "Yolanda, are you here? My baby, are you okay?" He ran from room to room in a panic.

Paul heard the shower running so he opened the bathroom door and screamed, "Yolanda, are you okay?" He wrapped his arms around her wet body and starting crying and caressing her. "My baby, I love you so much. What happened? I'd never forgive myself if something would ever happen to you. I can't live without you."

Paul kissed every inch of her body while she cried. They ended up—guess where—in bed and made passionate love. They sat up and talked for hours. Paul tried to convince her that he went to Europe on a business trip alone. At the last minute his wife insisted on going. Paul decided Europe would be a good place to ask for a divorce. The next day Yolanda came into the salon wearing a heart-shaped diamond around her neck, showing everybody what Paul had bought her in Europe. It was a belated Valentine's Day present.

"Lucy, look at my beautiful diamond. I told you Paul loves me. We're getting married as soon as the divorce is final. I'm so happy now."

"Yolanda, I think you're special and just a little naïve. I don't want to see you hurt anymore. Can I speak freely to you, as a friend?"

Lucille Fordin

"Yes. I trust your opinion."

"Calm down until you're sure the divorce is taking place. Cindy is certainly not acting like anything has changed in her life. From what I've seen and heard over and over again, ninety-eight percent of men never leave their wives."

"Lucy, I have to believe Paul loves me enough to leave Cindy. He loves me! Can't you just be happy for me?"

"Honey, if you're happy, I'm happy. I wish you all the luck in the world. I love you and I won't say another word to you. It's your life."

"Has Cindy been in to get her hair done?"

"And that's my business. Yolanda, you have to stop asking about Cindy." Yolanda's face dropped and in her next breath she said, "Please tell me."

"Okay Yolanda, while Paul was at your condo getting a blowjob, Cindy was also getting a blow from Renaldo." Yolanda started laughing, paid her bill and left. If she only knew that Cindy was telling Renaldo about their romantic trip to Europe and that Paul also gave Cindy a heart-shaped diamond. Real nice guy, a diamond for his wife and the same damned diamond for his girlfriend. He was a real smooth operator. I should say, real smooth ass! I've often wondered how guys like Paul can keep their stories straight.

The following Wednesday, the salon was quiet and I was exhausted from my ordeal with Yolanda. I decided to go out to lunch and left my receptionist Rosie in charge of running the salon. Rosie always takes care of the salon when I'm not there. When I returned, Rosie was in a panic. Both Yolanda and Cindy were in the salon. The shit was about to hit the fan.

Rosie said, "Lucy, what are we going to do? Cindy is getting a massage in Room One. I went to the ladies room for a second and when I came out I found out that Yolanda had come in asking for a facial. She's in Room Two!" I quickly ran to check on them and everything seemed quiet, but I could hear Cindy talking about her trip to Europe. Yolanda next door was talking about Paul. Only a curtain separated the two rooms. All I could think was, God help me.

Just then I heard a voice yell out, "Paul's a good man. If I were you, I'd marry him. My husband's name is Paul also, and we have a wonderful marriage!" Yolanda jumped off of the table and looked around the curtain. Cindy looked up and said, "See what my darling Paul bought me in Europe? I hope your Paul is as good to you as mine is to me."

Yolanda yelled out viciously, "He sure is! I have the same necklace you have." The two women examined the other's jewelry hanging from their necks, then simultaneously exclaimed, "We have the same necklace!"

"What a coincidence. My name is Cindy. What's yours?"

"Yolanda." Yolanda's eyes almost popped out of her head.

I was fit to be tied. As I entered the room, I said, "Girls, keep your voices down. This is not the place to air your dirty laundry. Cindy, I'm sorry this is happening. Yolanda, leave it go. Get dressed and calm down."

"You're not Cindy Artfield, are you?"

"Do I know you, Yolanda?"

"No, but you do now. Your Paul is my Paul." The pitch of Yolanda's voice went up high enough to break glass. There was dead silence. The veins were popping out in her neck. Cindy was speechless and didn't move a muscle.

"Cindy, did you hear me? Paul told me he told you he wanted a divorce, and in six months we're getting married."

All of a sudden Cindy came out of shock, and with rage in her voice she said, "I hear you, you little whore. I guess you're screwed, because I won't give him a divorce. He never asked me for a divorce and you definitely don't have the power to destroy my family. You're not the first whore he's had and you won't be the last. Now get out of here, you lowlife bitch."

You could hear a pin drop in the salon. Some people started laughing while others, like me, were in shock. I told everyone to get back to work and stepped in between Cindy and Yolanda.

"Yolanda, this isn't fair to me. Look at the two of you standing in your underwear and arguing. Please, for my sake and yours, just leave now."

But it was Cindy who quickly got dressed and stormed out. As Yolanda left, she screamed, "I'll kill that son of a bitch. I'm not a whore. She is."

Lucille Fordin

Who do you think Paul ended up with? Cindy went home and threw Paul out. Paul moved in with Yolanda. A month later Cindy wanted Paul back. He ran home with his tail between his legs and promised never to cheat again.

Yolanda got to keep the condo, the car, and all of the jewelry Paul had given her. I guess another marriage was saved, if you want to call it that.

We can all quite easily turn stupid when we're in love. Tough relationships can be harder than giving birth. The pain never seems to go away.

Chapter Three:
The Beauty Contestant and The Evil Eye

When I was three years old, I won first place in a beauty contest. I won enough baby food to feed the whole neighborhood for a year. An Italian lady living next door to us was so jealous because her daughter lost that she cursed me and tried to put the evil eye on my whole family. My Mom told me she called a priest for help and made me say prayers every night.

One day a beautiful Italian girl whose hair I had been cutting for four years came into the salon for her appointment. Margaret Ann was eighteen, a very tall, thin, gorgeous girl with a lot of insecurities. She had long, thick, black hair, big, round hazel eyes, puffy lips, and shapely legs that some of us could only dream of having. Who would think that someone as beautiful as this could be so insecure?

Margaret Ann had been in beauty pageants, one after the other, all her life. I was in the middle of cutting her hair when she looked up at me and asked, "Lucy, do you believe in the evil eye?"

"Yes, I most certainly do, but only if we are weak enough to let that evil into this world. You have to bestrong enough to fight away those evil feelings. I pray a lot at night, Margaret Ann. It helps me to sleep. Why are you asking? Are you having some problems?"

"Yes, I am. About six months ago, I entered a beauty contest and June, one of my competitors, started crying because she had lost. I took fourth place, so naturally I was upset too. She couldn't go to her mom for comfort because she would holler at her and embarrass her in front of everyone. Needless to say, I never liked the woman. She was a very mean person."

Lucille Fordin

Margaret Ann continued. "I put my arms around June, trying to console her, when May, her mother, walked in and said, 'Stop crying. You're making a fool out of me and you.' I should have minded my own business, I guess, but I couldn't help myself. I felt so sorry for June. Then her mother yelled at me, 'Take your hands off of my daughter.' May looked at June and said, 'You better stop crying right now. You will just have to practice more and lose five pounds. You're getting fat!'

"Just then my mom came running over and said, 'Don't you ever talk to my daughter that way, you witch. No wonder your daughter is crying. You are embarrassing her in front of all of these people. Lower your voice. You are making your daughter sick.'

"June's nasty mother replied, 'You're the witch, Ann. No one tells me what to do. I have given up plenty for this child. The least she can do for me is win!'

"June started crying and sobbing all over again and said, 'Mom I don't want to do this. I'm not good enough or even pretty enough to win." Then she fell back into my arms.

"May started screaming again. 'Take your hands off of my daughter. Get over here, you crybaby.' May pulled at her daughter like we were playing tug of war.

"My mom said, 'May, I've had enough of your obnoxious mouth. Don't yell at my daughter, you imbecile. I'll have you barred from all pageants for abuse. Let's go, Margaret Ann, this woman is crazy.'" Margaret Ann had tears in her eyes and started chewing her fingernails. As I looked up at her, the scissors snipped through my finger and I said, "Oops!"

Margaret Ann started crying. "Lucy, is my hair ruined?"

"No, Margaret Ann, but you have red highlights now. Let me get a band-aid and you get your hair washed. Then you can finish telling your story."

Margaret Ann was laughing on her way to the shampoo bowl. We both returned to my station and she continued her story. "As I got up, May raised her forefinger and baby finger and screamed in a crazy voice, 'I curse you and your whole family, especially your little princess.' I was so upset, I can't even remember everything she was screaming. She just kept cursing me as we left the pageant.

"On the way home, we got a flat tire and Mom went crazy. 'It's her curse,' she said. The next day I got a big pimple on my face. I stayed home from school two days because my cheek was so swollen. Mom said, 'It's the curse.' One of Dad's clients backed out of a big deal with him. Mom and Dad started fighting. Mom said, 'It's the curse.'"

When Margaret Ann started crying again, I stopped cutting her hair, while I still had fingers left. "Lucy, is your finger okay?" Yes, honey. I'll finish after you tell me the rest of the story. It's safer for you and me." Margaret Ann just smiled and continued talking.

"I fell and skinned my knee. My mom said, 'It's the curse.' So I said to myself, 'She might be right. What if it is the curse?'

"A month later I got very sick. I couldn't eat or sleep. I kept getting fevers. Mom and Dad took me to three different specialists and every doctor said there was nothing wrong with me. Mom was so upset she took me to our church to speak with the priest. Father John said, 'You can fight off the evil by praying.' So Father John prayed with us and said, 'Keep a positive attitude, dear. Wear your holy cross around your neck. These problems could be just incidental.' Mom asked Father John if there was a way for him to lift the evil eye from our family. 'There must be someone you can call to get us some help. Can you do an exorcism?'

'Ann, the church does not recognize exorcism. Take Margaret Ann home and I'll pray for you.'

"I felt much better for a while, but then I woke up with severe stomach cramps. I was rushed to the hospital and was given every test in the book. Dr. Dobson came into my room and said, 'Margaret Ann, have you had any trauma lately?'

'No, doctor,' I replied.

"Dr. Dobson turned to Mom and Dad and said, 'Maybe it's time to seek psychiatric help.'

"'My daughter is not crazy! Our family was cursed by a wicked Italian woman.'

"Dr. Dobson had a very puzzled look on his face. 'Mrs. Antinucci, I'm Catholic. I believe in medicine, but something strange is going on here. Only once in my career have I seen something like this before. Let me just ask, and this is off the record, do you know anyone who knows the special prayers to take the evil eye off someone? If you do, I suggest

Lucille Fordin

you call them now. You know, it can't hurt. These problems are not medical.'

"My mom remembered that her great grandmother who came from the old country believed strongly in the evil eye. I know my grandmother had a special prayer book to ward off evil.'

" "We don't even know what happened to my grandmother's prayer book when she died in Italy,' my mother said.

" 'I wish you luck,' Dr. Dobson said.

"After Mom made a hundred phone calls to every one she knew, she reached a cousin in Italy who said, 'Ann, you are a lucky woman. My best friend's grandmother, Maria, is in Florida visiting her family. Maybe she can help.'

"A week later the phone rang and a very old, weak voice said, 'I'm Maria. Are you Margaret Ann? I'm going to help you. Is your mother home? I never travel without my Grandma's prayer book. It was handed down to me because I am the strongest willed in our family. I can help you. I'm ninety years old and this could be very dangerous for me. The evil has to pass though my body to cleanse your family. It could kill me at my age, but I feel the need to help your family.' Maria chuckled strangely, 'How much longer can I live anyway?'

"The next day the old woman, dressed in a floor-length black dress, shawl and veil, came to our house. I was really scared. The minute Maria entered our house, she lifted her veil and her entire shriveled, wiry body started to shake. 'This is not good. I'm feeling a lot of evil here.' She let out a huge sigh. 'Bring the child to me. Ann, I need a bowl of water and some oil. Get my prayer book out of my purse.' Mom got everything Maria asked for. The old woman started pouring the oil into the bowl of water and we watched as the oil broke away into little balls dancing around the bowl.

"'Oh my God, this is not good. Everyone join hands,' Margaret Ann said, "Lucy, now I'm really scared. My hands are shaking.' Maria started reading prayers from her ancient prayer book. She was praying louder and louder until her whole body started shaking, and the sweat started rolling down her face. As she prayed, the oil stopped dancing in the bowl. It just would not go together like it was supposed to. The praying got louder as Maria's voice got stranger. Her voice started out normal, then almost became a scream, then turned into a deep man's voice.

Maria said, "Remove the evil from this child and this family. I implore you, in the name of the Father, and of the Son, and of the Holy Spirit, go back to where you came from.'

"Slowly the oil particles started moving closer together as Maria kept praying louder and more weirdly. After a few minutes the oil came together in one big ball. The old woman fell back into the chair and could not catch her breath. Her eyes rolled back in her head, and sweat was pouring from her body. Lucy, I thought she was dying. Mom ran fast for a glass of water. Dad was rubbing Maria's arm. Everyone was in a panic. All of a sudden Maria's eyes opened and she said, 'Bring me the child.'

"Maria, here I am," I said. The gasping, perspiring old woman grabbed me and started crying, squeezing me so tight that I couldn't breathe. 'You're free of the evil, child. Now go and enjoy your life. In the Name of the Father, the Son, and the Holy Spirit. Amen.'

"I couldn't believe it. I hadn't thought of my ailments since the old lady had arrived, and now I had no pains and I felt great! Everyone started crying, making the sign of the cross, and saying, 'Thank you, God.'

"Lucy, I believe Maria saved our lives from evil. I'm sure you must think I'm crazy."

"No, I don't think you're crazy, darling. I believe you. I believe in the evil eye. A lot of people believe in curses too. That's why so many of us wear these evil eye pendants around our necks to ward off the evil spirits. I'm glad you're okay, Margaret Ann, and that's all that counts. Maybe the next time you come for a haircut you'll tell me you're going to get married or something else as wonderful."

Margaret Ann started laughing and said, "Lucy, I'm too young to get married and Mom would really kill me."

Chapter Four:
Gina, Tina and Jekyll and Hyde

It was the end of March, and spring break, Easter and Passover were only a few days apart that year. The salon was very busy and our clients were very nervous because of the shopping, cooking and company they were expecting. My station was in the center of the salon, so I could hear and watch everything.

Spring break brings a lot of young adults to Florida. Some stay in hotels and some are lucky enough to have grandparents in condos to stay with.

Renaldo was an excellent Italian hairdresser. Gorgeous! The women loved him. His station was next to mine, and I loved to listen to his conversations.

Mrs. James was in Renaldo's chair, having her hair done, when I heard her say to him, "I'm exhausted. My granddaughter Gina is staying with me for two weeks. I love her dearly. Her girlfriend Pam is a nice girl too, but she sounds like a broken record sometimes. Look at this picture of Pam, Renaldo. She's little, cute and has too much hair. I'm afraid Pam's a little too loose to be with my granddaughter. I guess I won't get much sleep for awhile. Pam never stops talking from morning to night. I'd like to put a plug in her mouth!"

I had just finished my client and as I was walking through the salon, I heard someone say to me, "Hi Lucy." I was puzzled for a second and said, "Gina, it can't be you."

"It's me Lucy," Gina said with a big smile on her face. "I'm all grown up now. This is my girlfriend Pam. We're staying at Grandma's for two weeks, and we are definitely going to party!"

Lucille Fordin

The last time I saw Gina she was chubby, but only seventeen. She was twenty-one now, thin and beautiful. I looked at the two girls and said, "Party hardy, but try not to give your grandmother a heart attack." Gina and Pam giggled like two silly little kids.

"We're going to Coconut Grove tonight. Pam's boyfriend is meeting us and he's bringing a blind date for me. I hate blind dates, but I'm doing this for Pam. She's my best friend."

Pam tried to reassure Gina. "I'm sure Steve will bring someone nice for you. Steve's a cool guy."

"Pam, promise me you won't leave me alone with a strange guy."

"I promise, Gina."

"Girls, please be careful. Things can get a little wild in the Grove after midnight. I was your age once, and I made a lot of bad choices in men. When I think of it now, I'm very lucky to be alive. So have fun and try not to give your grandmother a nervous breakdown your first night here."

We all laughed and I said, "Be serious for a moment and listen to me. My mother always told me, 'If you are stuck in a bad situation, just get in a cab and come home.'"

"But Lucy, I'll have my grandmother's car. So if anything bad is about to take place, I'll run him over with the car and then I'll drive myself home."

I hesitated for a moment until I realized it was a joke. "Gina, make sure you hit him where it hurts the most."

"You mean crack his nuts!" Well, we started laughing and couldn't stop. We were literally crying. As I walked away I said, "Promise you'll tell me all about the blind date next week, and please be careful."

The following week I noticed Gina and Pam in the salon but they were not talking. They sat in the reception room with an empty chair between them. They both had sad faces. I knew something bad must have happened.

"Hi, Gina."

"Hi, Lucy."

I sat down between them and said, "Thanks for saving me a seat. Now I want to hear all about all the fun you're having on your vacation. Do I dare ask how your blind date went?"

Gina's eyes filled up with water, her head dropped down and the tears ran down her face. Pam immediately responded, "Not too good, Lucy. I'm mad at my boyfriend and Gina's still mad at me. The blind date was a real creep."

Pam started talking when very abruptly Gina said, "Shut up Pam. I'll tell Lucy what happened myself. Lucy, please promise me you'll never tell Grandma what I'm about to tell you right now."

"I promise, Gina."

"Saturday night we went to Coconut Grove and Pam's boyfriend Steve was staying with his best friend's brother for three days. When we arrived at the apartment, I was a basket case waiting to see what this guy looked like. As we walked up to the apartment, I made Pam promise she wouldn't leave me alone with this stranger unless I told her I felt safe.

"We knocked on the door and this gorgeous guy around thirty years old opened the door. 'Wow I hope you're Gina. I'm Gary, Steve's friend.' Pam ran in the door and immediately started kissing Steve. Gary seemed to be nice. So I said, 'Its nice to meet you, Gary.' He was mature and charming, so I knew I had to be cautious. I had no experience with older men. The oldest man I ever dated was twenty-four.

"We sat down and Gary brought us all beers. Within an hour I felt like I knew Gary all my life. He was fascinating. While he was telling me he was a stockbroker, I looked around the apartment. It looked like he had money. I didn't see any sign of a female living there. Gary told me he was divorced twice. Both of his wives were very jealous and he hated jealous women. I was uncomfortable because Pam was all over Steve, making out like crazy.

"Gary looked like he was ready to make a move on me when I said, 'Hey, what club are we going to? I'm ready to dance, let's go!" I suggested we take two cars.

'I promised Grandma I'd be home by 2am at the latest. You guys might want to stay at the club after we leave.'

"Gary grabbed my hand, smiled and said, 'We're going together, and I'll make sure we come home together. I'd never let anything happen to someone as sweet and pretty as you.' I immediately melted into dreamland and off we went to the club.

Lucille Fordin

"What a perfect gentleman Gary was. I kept thinking, 'Boy, could I fall in love with this guy.' A slow song came on and as we were holding each other on the dance floor, Gary was giving me one compliment after another. As he pulled me in closer and closer to his body, I could feel my heart pounding faster and faster. I couldn't stop thinking how stupid I was for being so scared.

"After a few drinks Gary asked me if I'd have dinner with him Sunday night. I jumped on it right away and said, 'Of course I will.'

"Around eleven thirty Pam said, 'Gina, we'll be in the park across the street. We just want to be alone for a little while. I promise I'll be back in an hour.'

"'Pam, you're drunk; please be careful. Are you sure the park is safe?'

"'Gina, you're such a baby, grow up. You worry too much. I'll be with Steve. He'll protect me. It's not like I'm a virgin or anything. I'll be fine.'

"After they left, Gary talked up a storm. He told me all about his life. I was fascinated listening to him. Guys my age rarely talk; they just want to get high and have sex. Gary was living a full and exciting life. I kept thinking, 'How could any woman want to give this man up? I could really fall in love with this guy.'

"It was now midnight and Gary asked me if I wanted something to snack on. All of a sudden he pulled his wallet out and said, 'Gina I'm so embarrassed, I left the rest of my money in my other pants at home.'

"I quickly replied, 'I have money, Steve.'

"'No thanks, Gina, I'd never let a beautiful women like you pick up the tab for me. It will take us only twenty minutes to get the money and come right back. Trust me, Pam and Steve won't be back for another half an hour to an hour.'

"Gary picked up my hand and said, 'You know you can trust me.' Gary talked so fast, before I knew it I followed him to the car. He was still being a perfect gentleman. So again I said to myself, 'Gina calm down, you're being stupid for being scared.' But I couldn't stop thinking that this guy is too good to be true.

"We talked all the way to the apartment and Gary assured me he wasn't seeing anyone else. There was nowhere to park in front so we had to go to the back of the building. He leaned over and put his lips on mine and then said, 'One day you'll be my wife.' I was speechless and felt a tingling sensation all over my body.

"'Gina, I don't think that it's safe to leave you back here by yourself. Please come in with me.' I hesitated but I didn't want to be alone in the back of the building either, so I went in.

"I sat down on the couch while he got his money. Then he came out and said, 'Gina I want you to stay with me tonight. I'm falling in love with you. I know you've got to feel something too.' Gary kept begging me to stay and I kept saying no.

"'Let's get back to the club before Pam gets back. You're moving too fast for me.'

"Gary said, 'Okay, you win, let's go.'

"Just then, Lucy, someone put a key in the door and pushed the door open.

"A short, cute girl walked right in and started screaming at Gary. 'You dirty son of a bitch, I'll kill you. Is this the whore you're cheating on me with?'

"Gary said, 'Tina, you're crazy, get out of here!'

"Tina ran toward Gary, screaming, 'I'm pregnant with your baby and you're fucking this bitch? I'll kill you.' I jumped off the couch and backed up until I felt the wall holding me up. I was shaking from my head down to my toes.

"Gary grabbed Tina by the arms and started shaking her, telling her to shut up. But she wouldn't stop screaming, 'You said you loved me. We were getting married. How could you do this to me? This is how you pay me back, by bringing your whore into my bed?' Gary smacked Tina right across the face.

"I was really scared. I had to get out of there, but my legs were frozen stiff.

"Tina ran in the bedroom and started throwing clothes all over the apartment, crying and screaming hysterically. 'Gary, I'm leaving so you can handle your own problems.'

"'No, you're not leaving. I'm leaving with you,' Gary said.

Lucille Fordin

"Tina just kept on screaming. 'See, bitch, I live here. These are my underwear and these are the rest of my clothes. I live here. You get out of here right now!'

"Gary pushed Tina into the bedroom and ran toward me. He tried to convince me he didn't love her and that he didn't know she was pregnant, that he had thrown her out the week before. 'Let's get out of here, Gina.'

"Just then Tina ripped the bedroom door open and ran after Gary with a broken bottle in her hand. 'You're not going anywhere with that whore,' she hollered.

"Gary grabbed the bottle out of her hand and smacked her right across the face! She fell down to the floor and didn't move. I thought he had killed her. I was shaking more than ever. Gary turned to me very calmly and said, 'Gina, let's go. I'll deal with Tina later.'

"I quickly said, 'You can stay and I'll go.'

"Gary grabbed my arm. With great force in his voice, he said, 'Gina, I want you, not her.' I was so nervous I forgot my car was right outside. All I knew was I had to get out of there fast.

'Gary, call me tomorrow and we'll meet for dinner, okay?' I would have said anything just to get out of there without getting hurt.

'Please, Gina, sit down a minute. I can't let you drive. You're shaking. I hope you know I'd never hurt you.'

"Then Tina started screaming again. 'Don't you believe that lying bastard. He told me the same thing. Can't you see the marks all over me from his beatings? Gary I love you, I'm carrying your baby. I'll never let you go.

Gary grabbed Tina and said, 'I told you to shut up, you witch.' He hit her so hard I couldn't believe it.

"He started shaking her; then he lifted her into the air like he was going to throw her down on the ground when I yelled out, 'My God! Put her down before you kill her!"

"Gina," I said in shock, "I would have done the same thing. How mad did Gary get after you yelled at him?"

"Gary turned to me with this cruel look on his face. 'This has nothing to do with you, Gina,' he said.

"I started moving closer to the door as Gary threw Tina on the couch, turned to me and said, 'Where do you think you're going?'

"Tina jumped off of the couch and pulled at Gary. 'You're mine. You belong to me. You're not going anywhere with that whore.'

"Gary hit her again and she fell to the floor. She didn't get up so fast this time. I took off like a bat out of hell.

"I was very angry with Pam. I started driving home when I remembered Pam and Steve, so I turned the car around and headed for the club.

"It was now one-thirty in the morning. Pam and Steve were nowhere in sight. I went across the street to the park and there the two of them were, sound asleep like babies.

"'Pam, Steve, wake up. We have to go.'"

"'Where's Gary?'

"'Don't even ask. A nightmare just took place at his apartment with somebody called Tina. I'll explain everything on the way home.

"'Gina, what actually happened? I need to get my clothes. Maybe you're over-reacting.'

"'Steve, I'm not over-reacting. I almost got hurt. Let's go now. Gary can ship your clothes to you. You can't go back there.'

"Lucy, the more I thought about Pam leaving me with that nut case, the madder I got."

"You poor thing! What an ordeal you went through. Gina, you and Pam are friends. Steve didn't know what Gary was really like. You were very lucky to escape without any injuries. What a creep he was! I'm so sorry this horrible experience happened to you. But listen, you're alive and Pam is still your best friend, so why don't you two hug and make up?" After a few seconds Pam and Gina started crying and apologizing to each other.

"Girls, I've had some bad experiences in my life and so has half of the world. Every experience in life is a lesson to make us smarter and more careful the next time."

Gina and Pam both jumped up and kissed me. They couldn't thank me enough for listening to them. "I'll see you two the next time you're in Florida. I have to get back to work before your grandmother suspects something. I should be going to the beach with you two so I could have some fun, but responsibility calls."

Chapter Five:
All My Children

It was the week of May 12th, Mother's Day. It was a very special time for our clients. Some were happy because their children were flying in, while some were depressed because of their inconsiderate children. I miss my mother the most on this day.

Mother's Day was a good time for me to show my appreciation to my clients. Mothers are very special, the hidden power of the world.

I had a beautiful buffet all week and the clients never stopped thanking me. The first client on Tuesday was just as important to me as the last one on Saturday evening. Seeing the smiles on the women's faces as they came into the salon was worth all the work I put into that whole week of parties. I went from happy to sad the following week.

Death and disaster never stopped. Seeing clients week after week, year after year, could make you feel like family. Sometimes feeling their pain and sharing their tragedies could make it very hard to get through a day.

Mrs. Cane came in and said, "Lucy, I have to catch a plane in two hours. Something horrible has happened. My granddaughter's house caught on fire. When her husband smelled the smoke it was too late. They couldn't save the house but they managed to get to a window. They were on the third floor. Her husband tried to get her to jump, but she wouldn't. He pushed her out the window. Thank God my granddaughter is alive, but something went wrong. Just as John was getting ready to drop the first child out the window for her to catch, the house exploded. All my granddaughter remembers is the three kids screaming 'Mommy, Mommy.' I'll never forget this Mother's Day present."

Lucille Fordin

Mrs. Cane was crying hysterically so I just held her in my arms. She was a good friend, not just a client of eleven years. Her granddaughter was in the hospital for six months or so. Three years later she met someone and fell in love. She ended up marrying and having two more children and a new life.

That same week, Mrs. Crane came in and told me her forty-eight-year-old son took the whole family skiing in Aspen Colorado for Mother's Day. Her son fell and broke his knee, but he was okay. The following week she got a call, and her son was dead! They started a lawsuit against the hospital after an autopsy determined a lump on his head had been overlooked.

Mrs. Crane said to me while I was doing her hair, "I'm rich. I don't need the money, and it certainly isn't going to bring my son back to me. I dropped the lawsuit."

She was under psychiatric care, and died shortly after our last conversation. The last thing I remember her saying to me was, "I still can't bear the pain. I just want to die." Two years later her husband died. I couldn't help thinking, "At least the family is together again."

The DiPietro's tragedy kept the entire salon depressed for three weeks. They were loved by everyone.

Samuel DiPietro was a very prominent lawyer. A few times a year he'd come to Florida to visit his parents especially for Mother's Day. The DiPietros had been coming to the salon for twelve years. Any time the family was in town they'd all come to see me. Jerry would show off her beautiful daughter-in-law along with her three beautiful grandchildren. What a nice family they were.

One day Jerry DiPietro came in and said, "Lucy, please get me in and out fast. We're going up North. My son is dead and we don't know what happened!" Jerry burst out crying and I held her in my arms. She looked at me and said she was told that her son killed himself.

My mouth dropped open and I said, "Jerry, I don't believe Sammy would kill himself. He was a strong, caring father, husband and son. I just don't believe it."

"I don't believe it either. He wouldn't do something like that to us or his family. Lucy, I just spoke to him yesterday and he was excited about settling a big, big case. He was planning on retiring. He was only fifty years old. His wife and kids are in shock and we're leaving in a few hours. Bill hasn't shown any reaction. He just doesn't believe his son is dead, and he won't rest until he finds out what exactly happened. We all want to know what or whose fault this is. We won't be back until we find out the truth!"

Three months later Bill and Jerry returned to Florida with an unbelievable story.

Every Sunday, their son Sammy and his family went to church and then went out for brunch. Sammy didn't feel well this particular Sunday so his wife and three kids went to church without him. When they returned, they found Sammy hanging in the hallway as they entered. They assumed he killed himself, until the investigation started. By then Bill and Jerry arrived. The autopsy was performed and they buried their son.

When the family left that Sunday, the front door was locked. When they returned the door was unlocked, which meant that Sammy had let someone in. After further investigation, it was learned that a man in a parked car was spotted out front, watching the house. Nothing was missing, so it couldn't have been a robbery. Sammy's arms had some bruising, and it couldn't be determined whether it was self-inflicted or not. It looked like he was forced to hang himself.

Sammy was always an honest lawyer. He was being investigated because one of his clients appeared to be laundering money for the mob, which made Sammy appear to be involved. He'd lose everything if he was, and the family knew nothing of it.

After settling a large case, Sammy had decided to retire. He was in the process of turning the rest of his cases over to another lawyer when he learned he had no way out. When Sammy found out that his client was in some shady business, he tried to drop him. He had built up his life's practice on being an honest, up-front lawyer.

The police detectives couldn't prove he was murdered, so they closed the case as a suicide. The family hired a private investigator. They were convinced that Sammy would never have killed himself.

The investigator learned that Sammy had taken on a client a year ago who was losing his business from mistakes a partner had made. The partner had just been arrested for embezzling one million dollars. The client was clean, but his partner wasn't. He was involved with the mob and had disappeared, never to be found again.

The responsibility fell on Sammy's client, which put Sammy in a bad spot because he liked his client and he had invested in the man's business to help prevent him from losing everything. When the business was successful again, the money that had been embezzled was owed to very shady people who wrongly held Sammy responsible for the one million-dollar theft.

Sammy obviously wanted out. He immediately sold his stock in the company and dropped the client. But evidently he was still being held responsible for the money. Nothing was ever proven; Sammy just ended up dead. That's all anyone knew, and then the case was dropped. The private investigator was told not to dig any deeper or everyone's lives would be at stake.

Jerry told me they didn't want to put the whole family in jeopardy because nothing they did would ever bring Sammy back. His family had plenty of money to live on, so they decided to leave things alone.

Jerry said, "The important thing is we know Sammy didn't kill himself. Everyone in the family was blaming him or herself for not noticing that Sammy was in trouble. Sammy didn't feel it was his responsibility to pay somebody else's debt. He was just in the wrong place at the wrong time. My only son is dead. I don't think Bill will ever be the same. I keep telling him we have to be okay for the grandchildren's sake, but I'm really worried about him."

Three months later Bill had a heart attack and had a triple by-pass operation. He is doing very well now. Jerry is so busy taking care of everyone she hasn't had time to even think about what happened. Some women are known to get stronger after something tragic happens. But when things eventually calm down, Jerry may start thinking about the past and could very well go into a state of depression. Only time will tell.

Chapter Six:
Condo Tragedies

The salon had experienced a lot of tragedy from clients in those past three months. I had to be strong even through I felt the same depression as my employees.

It was Thursday morning, and I decided that it was time to block out the bad and bring in some good. I put Y100 on the stereo. (Kenny Walker and Steve Young play the best music.) Before I knew it, everyone was happy and dancing to the music. I announced over the intercom that I was buying lunch for all the employees. They started cheering. I ordered my favorite consoling food- pizza, meatball subs and chicken wings. Nice and fattening, to fight depression. In between clients, the employees were eating, dancing, and thanking me for lunch.

All of a sudden, a client named Martha, who lives in a condo in Aventura said to me, "Give me a piece of pizza." I told Martha it was only for the employees. I couldn't give one client food without giving it to all of them. The bagels, cream cheese and coffee were for the clients. Martha was persistent.

"Lucy, I spend a lot of money in here, and you're too cheap to give me a lousy piece of pizza."

Zane, my hairstylist, came running over when he saw my disturbed expression. "Martha, I've been doing your hair for five years," he said, "and I won't let you talk to Lucy this way. She's too good to all the clients. She has food here all the time for you, and what about all the buffets for Mother's Day, Halloween and Christmas? Get your hair washed now and leave Lucy alone or I won't do your hair."

Lucille Fordin

Thank God, Martha shut up and had her hair washed. I thanked Zane and kissed him. We went in the back room and laughed until I was crying. Then Zane said, "Who do you want me to beat up now, Lucy?"

You could have heard a pin drop when Zane gave Martha her ultimatum. The clients were whispering and saying, "Good for him! She's a pain in the ass. I wish we could throw her out of her condo."

We had a great day and everyone was happy.

Friday morning came and the employees were showing up early for work, saying, "I couldn't wait to come to work and have more fun." The morning was light-hearted. After lunch I realized that Mrs. Cappy's daughter, Janet, failed to show up for her haircut.

"Rosie, please call and see why Janet didn't show up for her appointment."

"I will as soon as I have time. A lot of the women are coming in late because of a tragedy in one of their buildings. Someone jumped off their eighteenth floor balcony."

"Who was it?"

"No one knows yet. The women told me the area was blocked off and the police were everywhere." By the end of the day we found out that it was Janet Cappy who killed herself. Janet had a lot of problems.

Mrs. Cappy was a sweet, loving, gentle woman. Janet was her only child. Mr. Cappy had passed away five years ago, and now she was on her own.

A month after Janet was buried, Mrs. Cappy called for an appointment.

As soon as Mrs. Cappy entered the salon, I stopped checking the stock and ran toward her. "Mrs. Cappy, I'm so sorry for your loss."

"Lucy, where did I go wrong? I knew Janet was depressed, but I can't believe she killed herself. From the time her father died, she started drinking a lot and used it as an excuse. My husband had a very bad depression problem. After his stroke he didn't want to live, so he killed himself one night by overdosing on sleeping pills. Janet always believed we didn't do enough to help him. She also suffered from severe depression, but she wasn't depressed enough to kill herself."

"She moved out of my house five years ago. About three months ago she broke up with her boyfriend with whom she was living and moved in with me. She lost her job and never stopped drinking. She was seeing a psychiatrist. I thought she was doing fine but I guess I was wrong. A week before she killed herself she tried to go back with her boyfriend, but he wanted nothing to do with her. He told her she was crazy, like her father."

"Lucy, I was keeping a close eye on Janet, but when I went down to the laundry room to get the clothes, she just jumped. It's my fault; I shouldn't have left the apartment. I was only gone for five minutes. I didn't know what happened until there was a knock at my door. 'Do you have a daughter named Janet?' the policeman asked.

"'Yes, what's the problem?'

"The policeman said, 'Please sit down, I have something to tell you. Janet jumped from your balcony, and she's dead.'

"'What are you talking about? Janet is right here. I only left for five minutes to put the laundry in!' I started screaming for Janet. 'Janet, where are you?'

"Mrs. Cappy, please calm down. Janet is not here. I'm sorry, but she's gone.'

"Lucy, my life is over. I couldn't save my husband and now my beautiful daughter is dead. It's all my fault, I should have been able to save her!"

"Mrs. Cappy, it's not your fault. You had no way of knowing that Janet would do something like this.

"Lucy, Janet was a problem child. My husband always blamed himself because of his own depression problem. That's why we never had any more children. He made me use protection. Our sex life wasn't very good, but I loved him and that's all I cared about.

"A week before Janet died, she said, 'Mom, Daddy was here last night. He told me he loves me and misses me. He's lonely.'

"I figured it was the liquor talking. At night I could hear Janet talking in her sleep to someone. I called her psychiatrist and told him what was going on. He didn't seem to be too alarmed.

"Janet was on anti-depressants. Her boyfriend accused her of also doing drugs and acting very irrational. She was accusing him of cheating and she threatened to kill him.

Lucille Fordin

"I can't believe my daughter was so out of control. The police questioned me for hours until they realized I knew nothing. I never thought they were questioning me to make sure I didn't push her over the balcony. I didn't push her over the balcony. I just don't know where I went wrong. I might as well have pushed her because it's my fault.

"Mrs. Cappy, stop torturing yourself. It's not your fault. Maybe you should sell that apartment. It's only a reminder of the unpleasant things that took place there. Start a new life in a fresh place. Let me do your hair now and maybe you'll feel better."

Mrs. Cappy cried the whole time she was in the salon. A month later she put her condo up for sale but was having trouble selling the apartment. Finally she had a buyer and seemed to be doing well. She moved into her new condo in Boca Raton. I heard six months later that she died of a heart attack. She was eighty-three years old.

I believe Mrs. Cappy died of a broken heart. What a lovely lady she was. There's never an answer to "Why me?" Some people glide through life without ever experiencing such tragedy. Poor Mrs. Cappy had enough trials and tribulations for all of us. Tragedies never stop, but life is expected to go on.

The salon went from happy to sad again in minutes that Friday afternoon, after we heard about Janet's death.

Saturday morning, all the clients were talking about different tragedies that happened in their condo buildings. It was 8:00am and I was having coffee with six clients in the salon. The women showed up a half-hour early for their appointments to have coffee and bagels. Mrs. Dean said, "Did you hear what happened yesterday to Mrs. Cappy's daughter, Janet? I missed having lunch with my friend who lives in her building because that crazy girl killed herself. No one was allowed in or out of the building until the police investigated."

Our mouths dropped open in shock all at the same time and no one said a word until Mrs. Shane said to Mrs. Dean, "Lunch! All you can think about is lunch when a young girl is dead. What's wrong with you? I think you're crazy."

I wanted to smack Mrs. Dean in the face, but instead, I said, "Please, don't start fighting. I'm depressed enough."

Mrs. Shane said, "Lucy, you're too sensitive. I don't know how you run this salon as nice as you are to everyone. You need to toughen up. I'll tell you what happened six months ago in my condo building."

'I was watching TV when I heard fighting and screams coming from the apartment next door to me. Mr. Lowell, the owner, was out of town on business, so I thought it might be his family staying there. I heard things breaking and a lot of cursing. I called the security desk downstairs, and when they arrived, they found Mr. Lowell on the floor, passed out. He's seventy-eight and has heart trouble.'

'He came home from his business trip early and found his maid having sex with her boyfriend in his bed. Mr. Lowell thought there were burglars in his apartment. He was also having an affair with his maid. The shock was so great, Mr. Lowell passed out.'"

Mrs. Dean blurted out, "The old fool was smart. He took the maid, instead of the maid taking him. The last maid I had, I fired. My steaks kept disappearing from my freezer every time she cleaned my condo."

"I can top that story," Mrs. Conway said. "I live in a very expensive building where the cheapest condo is four hundred thousand dollars. A young couple bought the condo right above me, and one night, I heard a lot of crying. I had my terrace door open. It was January, and there was a wonderful cool breeze. I could see something flying around outside, so I went out on my balcony, and twenty dollar bills were flying everywhere. I picked up a hundred dollars on my balcony and the rest was flying through the air.

"A woman's voice was screaming, 'Your money's always been more important than me. I thought this would be a new start in a new condo, you lying, cheating thief. Now your dirty money's gone. Don't ever bring your drug money home again, or I'll throw you over the next time.'

"It got quiet for five minutes, and then I heard more screams. I ran out to the terrace again, and a man's voice said, 'I'll teach you a lesson, bitch. We'll see who throws who off the balcony.'

"I leaned over the balcony, in a dark corner, so they couldn't see me. The man was holding the girl by her feet over the balcony, fifteen floors up, saying, 'Are you ever going to touch my money again?' 'No,' she kept screaming, 'No, please don't drop me.'

Lucille Fordin

"I ran into my condo and called security. They were already on their way up to their apartment. They had three calls in a row complaining about the screams coming from the apartment above me."

We all said at the same time, "What did you do with the money?"

"Wait until I finish the story," Mrs. Conway said. "The next day, I found out that the couple wanted to spend a week in the condo to see if they liked the building. The owner of the condo was selling it on his own. He figured no one would know he let strangers in the building. Even with strict condo rules, people get away with certain things."

"Okay, Mrs. Conway, tell us, what did you do with the money?"

"I kept it, of course. I was awake all night. One night's pay. I felt like a hooker. Easy money. And besides, they were gone the next day. Finders keeper, losers weepers!"

I was feeling very down from all this negative talk, when Mrs. Marks said, "I can top that one."

I grabbed my head and said, "I can't take anymore. Please stop, ladies."

"Lucy, don't quit on us now. You'll love this story."

One by one, the women said, "Just one more." I told Mrs. Marks to tell her story.

She said, "Last year, my next door neighbor went to empty her trash. She opened the trash bin and her false teeth fell out. Down the garbage chute they went. It took three maintenance men all day to find her teeth."

We were screaming in laughter as the hairdressers arrived. I told the ladies to get their hair washed while I told everyone coming into the salon the story of the garbage teeth. Yuck!

Chapter Seven:
A Stiff Dick Has No Conscience

It was July and the rain wouldn't stop. The parking lot was flooded. Cancellations in the salon are normal when it's pouring. In Florida, a thunderstorm is like having five inches of snow up North. When you're retired, like sixty percent of our clients are, there's usually no reason to come out in the rain except to get your hair done. My hairdressers are forty to sixty years old, and experts in the trade. You might not be able to get another appointment in the same week if you cancel. Besides, the next day was the 4th of July and we would be closed.

The salon is black and white, very modern, and very clean. The black and white floor was getting slippery. The maid was running around like crazy, wiping up the puddles of water dripping from the umbrellas and raincoats. I didn't want anyone to slip, so I was on my hands and knees, wiping up water, too. The women kept coming. One woman's clothes had to be put into the dryer because she slipped and fell into a puddle. About ten pairs of shoes were drying under the hair dryers. I was helping another women take off her wet clothes when I heard someone say, "I gave up my third husband faster than I'll give up my hair appointment." I was moving so fast I felt like someone lit a firecracker under my ass.

I was glad to see Denise come in to have her hair cut and highlighted so I could take a break from all the confusion going on in the salon. Everyone was complaining, even the hairdressers. Like it was my fault it was raining.

I've been cutting Denise's hair since she was ten years old. She's eighteen now, and when Denise was only fourteen, her mother died. She was an only child, and she and her father were very lonely.

Lucille Fordin

As I was cutting her hair, I looked up at her and said, "Whose the lucky guy? You look like you swallowed a watermelon." I couldn't believe Denise was pregnant again.

Denise smiled and started laughing. One second later she had tears rolling down her cheeks from her pretty blue eyes.

"Lucy, I hate myself. I promised myself this would never happen again until I got married. Dad is furious with me. I didn't tell him I was pregnant until I couldn't hide it any longer. He kept saying to me, 'Denise you're gaining a lot of weight. Maybe you should go on a diet.' I just couldn't get up enough nerve to tell him. I didn't want to hurt him. I love my father very much, and I've put him through enough pain already. I kept thinking my boyfriend Dave would marry me, but instead he dumped me. I hate him."

"Denise I did your hair for your graduation and you weren't pregnant then. You should have used protection after getting pregnant when you were fifteen."

"You know, I was a virgin when I got pregnant the first time. I was stupid to think having a baby could ever take the place of my mother. That's why Dad made me give up the baby for adoption. He didn't want me to ruin my life over a mistake."

"Denise, I'm Catholic and abortion is against our religion. I know your father's a devout Catholic too, but as far as I'm concerned, he made the right decision for his daughter."

Denise started to cry again so I stopped putting her highlights in and put my arms around her. "Lucy, what am I going to do? Mom always liked you and I feel I can trust you."

"Denise, calm down and tell me what happened. Let's try and figure out an alternative. You're eighteen and the final decision has to be yours. What does your father want you to do? But most of all, what do you want to do?"

"Lucy, my heart tells me to keep the baby. Dad wants me to put it up for adoption like last time and have me go to college. Dave and his family want me to have an abortion. I abstained from sex after giving birth the first time . . . that is, until graduation night. The evening started out exciting and wonderful, but it ended up a sheer disaster.

"Dave picked me up in a limousine that night. It was a present from his grandfather. It was my first time in a limo, so I was very excited. I felt like Cinderella. We went to the dance and had a great time. After the dance, we went to a party at a friend's house and we continued to party the rest of the night. Everyone was sneaking outside to drink and do drugs. Dave tried to convince me that it would be a good experience for me to try some drugs. He literally forced me to try them. It was a big mistake for me. I had never smoked marijuana before.

"Dave was telling me how much he loved me and how after college we'd get married. We had been dating for six months. Dave was kissing me and started getting fresh. I told him to stop. He stopped immediately just like he always had in the past.

Everything was going great when I started to notice that Dave kept going outside with his friends, which I knew meant he was doing a lot of drugs all night. All of a sudden he said to me, 'Denise, you know I love you. How long do you think I can wait? If it's not you, it will be someone else. My hormones are out of control and I love you so much. Don't you trust me?'

On the way home in the limo he was all over me. He closed the curtain that separated the driver from us. He grabbed my breast, but it was different this time. A little petting here and there was different than grabbing. He was as high as a kite and wouldn't take no for an answer. Before I knew it, he was pulling off my underwear saying, 'Denise, I have to have it now. I can't wait any longer.'

"'No, Dave, please stop.' I tried pushing him off, but he just wouldn't give up. I said, 'I can't do it, Dave, please I can't get pregnant again!'

"Dave tried to reassure me that he'd be very careful. 'I'll pull it out in time. Nothing will happen. You're acting like a silly child.'

"I tried hard to push him away, but he grabbed my arms and before I knew it he had pushed it in me. Lucy, I lay there, looking at the stars through the moon roof, pretending this wasn't happening to me.

"Dave yelled out loud, 'I'm coming!'

"I was quickly brought back to reality and said, 'Dave, pull it out fast, please!' Dave looked up at me and pulled it out real fast. Semen shot all over me and the car. I thought I was safe. I was scared and very depressed."

Lucille Fordin

"Later, when I told Dave I was pregnant, he immediately said with rage in his eyes, 'How do I know its mine? I pulled it out in time. Get an abortion. I'll pay for it. I won't let you ruin my life.' Lucy, I could have killed him. I really thought Dave loved me. What am I going to do?"

"Denise, before you make a final decision, sit down and talk to your father. He loves you very much. Then maybe you should talk to a psychologist. After you're done thinking of all the responsibility that goes along with having a child, also try and think of what kind of life the child would have. When your head hurts from thinking too much, I suggest you go to church and pray to God and to your mother to help guide you through this difficult situation. I guarantee you, somehow, someday soon, the answer will come to you. It works for me every time. Whatever you decide to do, just promise me you'll talk to the doctor about birth control pills for your protection. You're a beautiful, sweet, sensitive girl, and you have nothing to be ashamed of. This happens to a lot of women. Sometimes men can be such animals. My mother use to say to me, 'Lucy, a stiff dick has no conscience.'

"Denise, we all have bad memories from our past. We have to learn to live with them just so we can survive in this world. I'm always here for you if you need someone to talk to." She thanked me over and over again for taking the time to listen to her.

A second after Denise left the salon, a client tripped over her own foot and dropped her bagel and coffee. It splashed another client and a cat fight began. It took fifteen minutes to calm the two women down and as I walked away, all I could think about was blowing them up for the 4th of July. The thought kept a smile on my face all day.

About three months later Denise came in the salon and looked like she was going to give birth any second. She was in good spirits.

"Lucy, I only want my hair trimmed one inch. The baby is due and I've decided to put it up for adoption. I'm going to college. I talked to the doctor and I'm going on birth control pills immediately after the baby is born. But someday I'll find my babies and bring them home."

"Denise, it sounds like you're happy with the decisions you've made."

"Yes, I am. Dad and I decided it would be better for the baby to start life with a mother and father who can give it a normal upbringing. Dad said, 'It's not fair for a child to grow up with a father who wants nothing to do with it or its mother.' And you know, he's right. It's not fair to ruin a child's life because of my mistake. Someday I'll find the right man, get married and have a beautiful family. I also promised myself some day I'll see my two children again."

I gave Denise a big hug and kiss. I wished her all the happiness in the world.

Denise had the baby and gave it up for adoption. Three years later she married a wonderful guy. I was invited to the wedding. She told me she told her husband everything and he promised her that one day he would help her to find her two children. Denise had one child with Paul and was pregnant with their second. Denise became a psychologist.

Two years later Denise came into the salon with three children. I was puzzled as I approached her. "Hi, Denise, who is this gorgeous little boy?" He looked around ten years old.

"Lucy, this is my son, Steven. Steven, say hi to Lucy. She's my friend and she'll be cutting your hair." While Steven was getting his hair washed, Denise told me the following beautiful story.

"Lucy, I'm so happy with Paul. Paul came home on Christmas Eve and said, 'Denise, I have a surprise for you.' Within a second, Dad came through the door with this gorgeous blond-haired, blue-eyed little boy. He said, 'I want you to meet my grandchild, Steven.'

"Lucy, I couldn't move. My body just froze in place. I started crying and couldn't stop. Dad said, 'Steven, this is your mother.' I opened my arms and Steven ran to me like we had never been apart. I'm so happy."

"Paul and Dad found Steven in a foster home. He was very sick as a child so no one would adopt him. Dad and Paul tried to find my daughter, but had no luck. One day I'll find her. I'll never stop trying, but for now I want to enjoy Steven to the fullest."

Three years later Denise found her daughter Joanne, who also ended up in a foster home. Her adoptive parents were killed in a car accident. They were drug addicts.

"These children have had a lot of grief, and I'm responsible, but now they'll have a beautiful, loving family who will always be there for them. Always."

Lucille Fordin

I wish everyone's tragedies could turn out this way. I know people who have been looking for their children for years and still can't find them. Raising children is never easy. It becomes an instant on-the-job training experience. Children think they know it all. Don't dare try and tell them something or what to do. But they're in great need of a voice of authority. The world would be a mess if everyone ran around doing what they wanted. Everyone needs some direction. If not, life would be one big boring siesta.

I went back to being a boss. Mrs. Keller came in looking like a drowned rat. Forget her wet clothes, I thought. I'd better throw her whole body in the clothes dryer.

Chapter Eight:
Having Your Cake and Wearing It Too

It's Saturday. Family day. Our younger clientele like the high style precision haircuts and the fashionable colors. Their parents, on the other hand, have a different idea of what their children should look like: old fashioned. There's always lots of arguing going on between the parents and their kids. Oh my God! One kid just threw a handful of rollers on the floor and at the same time another child bumped into one of my top hairstylists, Gigi. She slipped on a roller and went down, taking the child with her. Gigi was on the bottom and the kid was on top of her. I thought she was dead. Neither one had a scratch. The parents never even apologized for their children and told Gigi to be more careful. What a joke! I ended up in the bathroom almost choking to death from laughter. It was a Candid Camera moment.

Saturday brought a lot of tension because the hairdressers were tired from the week. I needed the strength of King Kong to keep everyone going, along with taking care of my clients and the rest of the salon.

Gigi was one of my busiest hairdressers. She loved her work and did an excellent job. She was a bombshell! Her client was throwing a fit. She was one hour late, so I quickly stepped in and offered to apply the color on her hair.

I am an expert colorist. It took me years of training to be able to look at anyone's hair and mix the proper color. But in this case, Gigi had the woman's formula.

When I finished putting the color on Gigi's client, my next client was sitting in my chair, a very wealthy twelve-year-old girl. Her family came from old money. I couldn't help but think how lucky this child was, being

Lucille Fordin

dropped off in a limousine while her nanny waited for her. The outfit she was wearing cost more than I make in a week.

"Hi, Samantha, how do you want your hair cut today?"

"Lucy, I only want a trim. I don't want my hair cut short. Only half an inch. I'll measure it later."

"Samantha, forget about measuring your hair and tell me how school is going."

"School is fine, but Lucy, Mom doesn't love me."

"Samantha, why do you feel that way? I've been doing your mom's hair for nine years and all she ever talks about is how much she loves you. She always mentions you and doesn't hesitate to say how proud she is of you. Maybe I can help. Would you like to tell me what's wrong?"

"All my friends have work to do around the house and get an allowance. Every time I ask my mom if I can help, she tells me we have servants to do the work. She will not let me do the things my friends do to earn money. If I want money, she just gives it to me."

"Samantha, learning to live with a lot of money can in some ways be just as hard as having no money at all. I know what you mean. I remember feeling the same way, but we were poor."

"What did you do, Lucy?"

"One day I said to my mother, 'You don't love me. All of my friends have chores to do around their houses, but you won't let me. You keep telling me, "Lucy, you'll be doing dishes the rest of your life. I don't want you doing them now. Just go out and have fun."'

"Samantha, my Mom thought she was doing me a favor until I told her how I felt. Our parents only know what's on our minds if we tell them. I was always told that the rich marry the rich and the poor marry the poor. I wish I had had servants like you. My mom had to work like a dog in our home. She had no choice. Your Mom is rich, and you'll have a much easier life than most. If you really want to learn how to do housework, you could always ask the servants if they would show you some of the things they do. I think you should go home and tell your mom everything you told me. You'll be surprised. I think she'll understand."

"Lucy, did your mother let you wash dishes once you told her?"

"Oh, yes she did, and boy, was I sorry I opened my big fat mouth."

Samantha started giggling and asked me, "Why were you sorry?"

"I was washing dishes for three months and Mom would say, 'Lucy, you're doing dishes because I love you, not because I want you to do them.' So I said, 'Mom, could you please love me a little less?'"

Samantha laughed and promised me she would talk to her mom.

I try to be very careful when I'm talking to children. They can be very easily misled or swayed in the wrong direction. I can only hope that I give them the right advice.

It was now 1:00 on Saturday afternoon, and I was wishing it was Sunday when I heard, "I want my manicure now." I quickly ran over to the client and asked if she would like to use one of the other manicurists. Her girl was only a half-hour late.

"Mrs. Swane, let me get you some coffee and a bagel. It won't be a long wait."

"My money is good anywhere. I want my manicure now."

I wanted to knock her down and tramp on her face, but instead, being the lady I am, I had another manicurist take her immediately. As I walked away, I noticed Jennifer in the waiting area. Jennifer was a very trusting, nice girl, a little over-weight, but very pretty, with big, piercing green eyes that sparkled in the sunlight. Her mother constantly told her daughter that she was prettier than her child could ever be, and that Jennifer needed to lose some weight.

When Jennifer was sixteen she found her mom kissing her teenage boyfriend on the lips in their kitchen. Jennifer broke up with him immediately.

Her mom blamed it on the boy. She said, "He kissed me first. I didn't do anything wrong. I love you."

Jennifer repeatedly told me in the salon, "I hate my mother. She's a whore."

Her mother used to say, "You can't keep any man happy. That's why they want me. You're jealous of your own mother."

Her mother was a real creep in my eyes. Mothers are supposed to give us strength, show us the right path to follow, and give us lots of encouragement. Trust is a big factor.

Jennifer wanted out of her house so badly, but she never made enough money to move out. At eighteen she fell in love and married just to get out of the house.

Lucille Fordin

Jennifer was six months pregnant when she came to the salon to get a body wave and haircut. While I was rolling her perm, she said, "Hi, Lucy I'm so happy with Bob. He's my whole life. He's a good husband and I'm sure that he'll make a good father. We're very happy together."

"Jennifer, I'm so happy for you. I can't wait till the baby comes."

"I'll never do to my child what my mother has done to me. We're better friends now than we ever were before. I don't have to worry anymore because Bob loves me, and only me."

"Jennifer, I can't wait to start buying baby gifts for you. I've never seen you so confident about your life."

"Lucy, I took the day off from work to get my hair done. Dad is out of town. Mom called and said she was lonely. I told Bob I would meet him at Mom's for dinner around six, so you have plenty of time to do my hair. I wish I could get my hair done every week. I just love talking to you, Lucy. You have helped me in so many ways."

I had Jennifer finished by four-thirty.

"Lucy, my hair looks beautiful. It was time for a change. I can't wait until Bob sees the new me. I feel great. I'm on my way to Mom's now, so I'll see you soon."

The next day Jennifer called me at the salon, crying hysterically. "Everyone hated my hair," she said. "Do you have time to change it? I just want you to cut it real short."

"Jennifer, please come in."

Jennifer was at the salon practically before I hung up the phone. She was still crying.

"My hair is ruined. I hate it. I want it off. I want my head shaved bald!"

It took me an hour to calm her down. "Jennifer, I'll cut your hair short, but I refuse to shave your head. You're hurting my feelings. I'd never ruin your hair or do anything to upset you. I have clients who moved to Boca Raton and Deerfield Beach who still come to me for their perms. One thing I know is that my work is good. I like you very much. When you left here, you were in love with your hair. What happened to make you want to shave your head?"

"I hate my mother and I hate Bob. I don't want anyone to ever look at me again. I want my head shaved now!"

"Okay, Jennifer, I'll cut your hair short first, and if you don't like it, then I'll shave it for you. You're beautiful and you're not acting like the Jennifer I know."

Jennifer started crying and apologizing like crazy. Then it all came out.

"Lucy, I'm so sorry. I didn't mean to hurt you. I just feel like I want to die! I won't let my child come into this sick world. My mother's a whore, and I threw Bob out. I'll never be with another man again in my life."

"Oh no, not again! What did your mother do to you this time? What did Bob do to make you so sick? Can't you try and work things out for the baby's sake? It can't be that bad, can it?"

"It's bad, Lucy, real bad. After you did my hair, I couldn't wait for Mom and Bob to see me. I looked beautiful and felt great. I stopped at the bakery and bought a cake because I was done early. Bob loves carrot cake and Mom never has dessert.

"Mom said, 'You're fat enough, Jennifer, you don't need dessert.' I'm pregnant mother, not fat. I got it for Bob because he likes dessert after dinner. So that's why it's here!"

"When I was parking my car I noticed Bob's car, which meant he got off work early. I was an hour early myself and couldn't wait for them to see my hair. I grabbed the carrot cake and hurried in. I was so excited until I opened the front door. Bob and Mom were on the couch stark naked, having sex! I stood there with my mouth wide open in shock, while the two of them scrambled to put their clothes on.

"Jennifer, I'm really sorry. What did they say?"

Bob started apologizing and blamed Mom." He said, 'She started kissing me. It's been a long time since I've had any sex. You're always sick. I didn't mean it. Please, it will never happen again! It was a big mistake.'

"'Mom, how could you do this to me? Haven't you done enough to me already? I hate you! You're a whore! How could Dad live with you, or doesn't he know that you would screw the whole world if you could? I'm telling Dad. This time you have really put the icing on the cake. I don't ever want to see you again!'

Lucille Fordin

"'Stop acting like a child, Jennifer,' my mom said. 'Had you satisfied Bob, he wouldn't need a real woman like me. You're just jealous. I did you a favor. This way Bob didn't have to find someone else. I protected him for you. You should be thanking me instead of being mad at me. And what did you do to your hair? It's not bad enough that you're fat, but now you look like a pickaninny. No wonder you can't keep a man.'

"Bob was begging me to forgive him and Mom was laughing at me. Lucy, I took that carrot cake and I smashed it over Mom's head and left."

Jennifer laughed hysterically. "You should have seen her standing there with the cake all over her face and head. That was all she was wearing." Jennifer started crying again.

"I'm so sorry. You're such a good girl. I just don't know why this is happening to you. But you'll survive. Your best bet is to stay away from her. That mother of yours has some serious problems. She's a very sick woman. Are you going to tell your father?"

"I want to, but I don't want to destroy his life either. What if he doesn't believe me? I've never told him anything about all of this. I've always felt that he'd find out for himself."

"What happened with Bob after you went home?"

"He showed up about an hour later. He said he waited to give me time to calm down, and he kept begging me not to leave him. He said he made a terrible mistake and would never have anything to do with my mother again."

"'Your mother seduced me,'" he said.

"I told Bob I didn't want anything to do with him and I made him leave. Lucy, now that I have calmed down a little, I really want my hair cut short. My hair is reminding me of what happened."

"I guess you're right."

I cut Jennifer's hair real short. She looked adorable. She promised me she would get some kind of counseling. I told her to call me day or night if she needed someone to talk to, and then I kissed her good-bye.

A few days later I called Jennifer to see if she was okay. She was thinking about taking Bob back. Her counselor convinced her that her mother was a sick individual and needed a lot of help.

One month later Bob and Jennifer were back living together. Jennifer's baby was due in approximately two weeks. She seemed to be doing pretty well. She never told her father what happened. I guess the pain was too much for this sweet girl to handle because Jennifer ended up killing herself and the baby. She thrust a knife into her stomach and bled to death. A note was found by her side. It read:

"I will not let my child live through
the pain I've suffered from this world.
I'm taking my child with me to a new
world. I want my friends to know that
I will be very happy now.
      Love, Jennifer."

When things like Jennifer's nightmare happen it always reminds me of what my mother use to drill in my head time and time again: "Time will heal all wounds. You must stay strong." Some are lucky with their lives, while some are not so lucky. I had a lot of trouble fighting off the depression I felt for Jennifer. Her mother didn't deserve to live.

Chapter Nine:
One of the Best Kept Secrets I Ever Heard: from a $500 Pee to a Law Degree

Molly Smith was raised in a family with a lot of secrets. She was fifteen when her mother threw her out to live in the streets because her mother was convinced that Molly was a liar and trying to ruin her life. Her father worked in construction. Her mother was a waitress and worked until 2am, five nights a week.

It was Wednesday, a slow day. I was feeling very homesick when I heard Rosie, my trusted receptionist, say over the loudspeaker, "Lucy, please come to the front desk. A friend of yours from Pittsburgh is here to see you." I immediately stopped checking my stock and ran to the front desk. I didn't recognize the young woman for a minute. As I got closer, I realized it was Molly Smith. I put my arms around her and gave her a big kiss on her cheek.

"How is your sister Jan? We had so much fun in high school. I still remember taking you to McDonald's for a cheeseburger and fries. Jan would say to you, 'Molly, there's a cute guy.' You would immediately raise your little hand and wave, and the guys would wave back to us. They couldn't resist your cute little face. You were so beautiful, Molly, and you're still beautiful. Your skin is like butter. I always knew you would grow up to be a knockout. Why don't you let me cut off your split ends and we can catch up."

"Lucy, the shop is beautiful and I do need to get my hair cut. I'm starting a new life in Florida. I'm either working or going to school and I never have enough time for anything else."

Lucille Fordin

While Molly was getting her hair washed, I was wondering why every time I mentioned Jan her eyes would start to mist up and for a second a very sad look would come over her face.

"Molly, let me take two to three inches off. Your ends are really dry and split."

"Yes," she said without hesitation.

"Now you can tell me all about Pittsburgh. Is Jan married? I haven't seen her in eight years. The last I heard from my sister Roxanne was that Jan was having some kind of problems and was in the hospital for some kind of treatment."

Molly's eyes filled up with water and said, "Jan is dead. She killed herself."

I was in shock and cut my finger with the scissors.

"I'm sorry, Lucy," Molly said, "I didn't know you had no idea about Jan. I thought for sure everyone knew about it. It was the talk of the town forever."

"Molly, I was Jan's best friend and I want to be your friend too. There's nothing you can tell me to make me ever stop loving Jan or you."

Molly took a deep breath and, with tears in her eyes, told me the story of her sister's death.

"Well, you know Mom always worked at night. She and Dad got drunk together on the weekends. That was the only time they spent together. Jan cooked dinner every night and took care of me. Some nights Dad would get very drunk and start screaming at us and calling Mom a whore.

"Jan would put me to bed every night and promised me she would never let anyone hurt me or she would kill them. Dad always said to Jan, 'You're my special girl.' I always thought he loved her more than me.

"One Wednesday night, Dad came home drunk. I was in bed and could hear Jan and Dad arguing. Jan was crying when she came in to bed. Every time I would mention to Jan, 'Wouldn't it be nice if we had our own bedrooms?' she would say, 'I'll never leave you alone in this house, Molly. Some day you will understand.'

A client came out of the ladies room and said, "Lucy, the bathroom is flooded." I excused myself for a minute and ran for the plunger. It was the maid's day off and water was everywhere. I wasn't glad I had a flood, but it gave me a few minutes to contain myself. I took a deep breath and went back to my chair.

"Molly, you have such pretty, long blonde hair." She smiled, then a sad look came over her face. "Fighting every night became a ritual between Jan and Dad. Then on the weekends when Mom was home, everything would be just fine."

"When Jan was graduating from high school, Dad told me I would be his special girl now that Jan was bad and wouldn't listen to him anymore. I was excited because I thought it meant Dad loved me as much as Jan.

"One night after dinner, Jan said, 'Molly, go in your room and do your homework. I have to go food shopping. I'll be back in one hour and I'll bring you an ice cream. Promise me you'll stay in your room and do your work quietly. Dad passed out and I don't want you to wake him.'

"I promised Jan I wouldn't leave my room and I would be done with my homework by the time she got home. One hour after Jan left, Dad woke up and said to me, 'Molly, where's your sister? She probably snuck out to see a boy. She's a whore just like her mother. You're the only one who loves me. Come into my bedroom and we'll watch TV.'

"'Dad, I promised Jan I would finish my homework. She went shopping.'

"'Molly, you're twelve years old. Don't you have a mind of your own? I love you more than Jan. Please come watch television with me. I'm lonely.'

"'I told you, Dad, I will be there in five minutes. I only have a few more things to finish and my homework will be done.'

"I did my work as slowly as I could, hoping Jan would come home. I hated the smell of liquor on Dad's breath. He stunk like a dead rat. I finished my homework and went into Dad's room to watch television.

"'Come over here, Molly. Come close to Daddy and lie on my lap.'"

"While Dad was rubbing my head and telling me I was his special girl, the front door opened and Jan started hollering. "'Molly, where are you?' She opened the door to Dad's bedroom, grabbed me and sent me to my room with the ice cream she bought me. I could hear Jan and Dad fighting and screaming at each other.

Lucille Fordin

"Jan told Dad, 'If you ever touch Molly I'll kill you. I'm telling Mom what you did to me. You're a drunk. I'm not special to you. I know now what you did to me was sick. You're a demented human being and should be put away for what you did. I'm warning you now, don't get near Molly again. I hate you!'

"Finally I said, 'Jan, you're just jealous. He told me I'm going to be his special girl because you don't listen to him anymore.'

"'Look, Molly, I love you. I'm only protecting you.'

"'Why do you think you have to protect me from Dad?'

"'You don't understand. Let me ask you, did Dad ever try to touch you anywhere on your body?'

"'Jan, are you okay? Dad would never try anything like that. He loves me.'

"'Molly, it's time for me to tell you something, and I want you to listen to me very carefully. You're almost thirteen and I have never told anyone what I'm about to tell you now, not even Mom. Dad is an alcoholic. When he drinks too much, he forgets I'm his daughter. It all started when I was nine. Dad found out Mom was cheating on him. Dad made me his special little girl. One night after I put you to sleep, Dad came in the room and said to me, "Jan, come watch TV with me. I'm lonely. Your Mom is never home."'

I finished cutting Molly's hair, took a deep breath and listened to the rest of the story.

"'I would lie in bed with Dad and he'd rub my head and tell me how special I was. Pretty soon Dad started touching me all over. Then he would make me touch him. He told me all fathers do these things with their kids, and I believed him.'

"'As I got older, I found out it wasn't normal for a father to have sex with his daughter. I wanted to tell Mom so badly but I didn't think she'd believe me. The only reason I stay here is to protect you. I knew if I gave him what he wanted he'd leave you alone. Now I see the same thing starting to happen to you. Don't you ever let Dad touch your body. When he's drunk he can't control himself. Molly, please don't ever lie to me. You tell me if something bad happens. Promise me you won't tell anyone what I just told you. He has been warned. Do you understand what I'm telling you?'

"'Yes, I understand.'

"One month later, Jan and Dad got into a terrible fight over the advances Dad was making toward both of us. We refused to go to his room. This time Dad smacked Jan right across the face and said, 'You're a whore just like your mother.'

Jan said, 'I'm telling Mom, you son of a bitch!'

"Dad passed out and Jan and I sat and talked until Mom came home. Mom sat in between us and Jan told her everything. At first it looked like Mom believed Jan, but then she started yelling at Jan.

"'There's no way that I wouldn't have sensed something like this. How could you say your father touched you? He wouldn't do something that horrible. I'm taking you to a psychiatrist. I don't want to hear another word about this again, you hear me?' Jan was put in a hospital for a month. When she came home, she never mentioned what happened again. She got a job and refused to move out on her own."

"Molly, Jan stayed to protect you," I said. "She felt her life was ruined. All she could do was try to protect you."

"Lucy, Jan and Mom were always fighting. One day Mom told Jan to leave, but Jan wouldn't. I had to tell her my secret. I told her that Dad had molested me twice. The only thing she said was, 'Nothing matters now.' She was in a deep depression."

"Jan moved into a studio apartment and had a decent job, but she was never the same after that. Eight months later she overdosed on sleeping pills and killed herself. We found her lying on the couch; the apartment was destroyed. On the floor was an empty bottle of scotch and a baseball bat.

Molly started crying and twirling her hair around her finger. "It's my fault."

"Molly, let me get you some water. Honey, it's not your fault." I ran for the water. I was so nervous and upset I didn't know what to do.

When I returned, Molly was still sobbing. "When I turned fifteen a year later, my father tried to molest me again," she said. "That's when I told Mom.

"She said, 'You can't possibly be my child. Get out of here, you liar. You're a whore just like your sister was.'

"I left home and went to live on the streets. I miss Jan so much."

Lucille Fordin

"Molly, I am so sorry. I can't believe what you've been through and what happened to poor Jan. This was one of the best kept secrets I've ever heard."

"I'm doing good now. I'm studying to be a lawyer. I became a pretty good prostitute while I was trying to survive the streets. I had no choice. I tried everywhere to get a job, but I didn't have a diploma."

"Molly, stop blaming yourself. It wasn't your fault. You're a beautiful girl and very intelligent for someone who hasn't graduated from high school. I remember you making straight A's in school."

"Lucy, I have everything figured out. I'll take the test to get my GED, then I go to college to become a lawyer. I have to do this for Jan. This was my dream and I made myself a promise that I would make something out of my life. I'll keep in touch with you to let you know how I'm doing."

"Molly, here's my phone number at home. Call me anytime. I know you'll make it. We Pittsburgers are strong-willed people. Look at me. I fulfilled my dreams. I own my own salon and I'm even a pretty good plumber. Anytime you need a friend, I'm here for you. Think of me as family."

Two months passed and Molly came in the salon with good and bad news. The good news was she had gotten her high school diploma and had enrolled in college. The bad news was, with the help of some influential clients, she was putting herself through college by being a prostitute.

Molly was going to school all day and turning tricks all night. I spoke to Molly at least once if not twice a month for the next year, and she was happy and content. She tried job after job but couldn't make enough money to pay for her college classes. She promised me that when she made enough money to pay for college she would never sell her body again. She said she'd be very careful. I could only hope for her sake that she meant what she said.

Six months later when she came in the salon for a haircut, she told me the following unbelievable story "Lucy, I know I told you I'd never tell you about my johns, but this one is very funny. Can I tell you about this one rich guy that I see once a month?"

"Sure, Molly, tell me. You know you can tell me anything. I think I can handle it."

"I have thirty regular men that I see. Once a month I have a john who pays me five hundred dollars a night. All I have to do is put on a lace body suit and dance to a sexy song of his choice. I'm not allowed to touch him. He lies on the floor naked, and I dance all around him as his penis gets harder and harder until he looks like he's ready to explode.

"After half an hour of him masturbating and watching me dance, I walk over to him, straddle his body, talk dirty to him, and then . . . I piss all over him! He reaches his climax when the warm piss runs all over his penis. The only thing that runs through my head is, 'Piss on him, piss on him good.'

My eyes and mouth opened wide and we burst out laughing for ten minutes. I couldn't believe that someone would pay another person five hundred dollars to piss on them.

Molly quit being a prostitute the day she graduated from law school. At the beginning she took on plenty of charity cases, especially the ones involving children. She was on a mission to help as many children as she possibly could, remembering her own troubled childhood.

She lives a perfectly clean life now. She's married and has two beautiful children. She told her husband the truth from the very beginning, and we never mention the horrible past she lived. I know this might sound strange, but I give Molly a lot of credit. She had a goal and once she reached that goal, she went on with her life and never looked back.

Of course Molly was lucky that she never got hurt. Her johns were all rich and well-connected men who needed her special attention. To turn out the way she did, making something beautiful out of her miserable earlier life, was definitely an accomplishment. Too many prostitutes either end up dead, very badly beaten, or killing themselves because they can't live with themselves for who they are, what they have done and the hand life has dealt them. Then there's the possibility of disease and drug abuse. It's true, only the strong survive.

Chapter Ten:
Big Bananas Foster

One day in August a very sexy barmaid named Dawn came into the salon for highlights. She was gorgeous. Dawn had long black velvet hair with red highlights, hazel eyes and a tall, lean body with legs that wouldn't quit. Dawn had a rough life as a child. She was very poor and had to learn to fend for herself. She was very good at sports.

"Hi Lucy, I need my hair colored. I met a great guy named Steven Parker and I plan on having him for dessert tonight after dinner."

"Dawn, is he a cream puff or a Bananas Foster?"

"Oh, definitely a big Bananas Foster!" We giggled like little girls.

"Dawn, get your hair washed and change your clothes. I'll meet you at my station."

Every color job is done differently. I put her highlights in on wet hair to slow down the bleaching process, bringing up the highlights one stage before the red is applied. A magnificent glow appeared throughout her hair.

"Okay, where did you meet Steven and what does he look like?"

"I met him at Joe's Tavern after work where a bunch of us go to unwind, eat, have a few drinks, and shoot some pool."

"One night I walked up to the pool table, laid my money down and said, 'I'll play the winner.' 'I made eye contact with a tall blond guy with piercing blue eyes. It was strange but I felt tingles in my body. I said to myself, What the hell is this I'm feeling?

"I felt the need to prove I was a tough girl, which is hard when you're a loving, sensitive kind of girl. I was mush inside, but I tried not to show it. I played to win, and I did. So Steven asked me to have a drink with him. He was laughing and making jokes to everyone about losing to a woman. I remember thinking, Wow, he's good-looking and a good sport.

"I've always hated sore losers. They make such fools out of themselves. That's one thing I tried never to do. I hate to be embarrassed. I've always figured, if I'm nice, I'll get treated nice. Lucy, you know, that I don't have a mean bone in my body. I live for love. Feeling love is so rewarding. It's a shame people don't know that it takes much more energy to hate than it does to love.

"Steven walked me to my car and said, 'Would it be okay if I kissed you?' I said, 'Sure.' Our lips met and I felt something that I never felt before. The kiss was soft and gentle, and my whole body was tingling. I had heard stories of these things happening to other people, but it never happened to me before. People say you always know when you're in love, but you really don't know the feeling until something like this happens. Love is wonderful. Oh, but it can also be a curse."

"Dawn, I'm happy for you."

"Lucy, this is the first time I could say I really know what making love is. Steven waited till I felt comfortable. When I was ready, he was so gentle. I felt like I died and went to heaven. After a couple of months I started asking Steven if I could see his apartment. I wanted to see where and how he lived. It just seemed funny to me that he always had an excuse as to why we couldn't go there. For instance, he would say, 'My friends are staying over,' or 'The place is a mess.'

"After three months passed, Steven said, 'How about spending the weekend at my apartment? I want to be with you day and night, Dawn. I'm in love with you.' Well, you know I immediately said, 'Yes.' Tonight's the night, Lucy, so please make me beautiful, and wish me luck!"

"Your color is beautiful. Should I trim your hair?"

"No, Lucy, I'll be back in a few weeks for the trim so I can tell you what happens."

"Good idea," I blurted out. "You go, girl, and make sure you have a double helping of your big Bananas Foster!"

Six weeks went by, I couldn't wait to hear about her love affair with dessert boy. Once I knew Dawn was coming in the salon, I couldn't get through the day fast enough. It was a Friday evening around 6:00, and I felt like Barbara Walters waiting to get a story. The salon was quiet; almost everyone had gone for the day

"Hi, Lucy." Dawn entered the salon, looking as if her dog has just died.

"Hi Dawn, what's wrong? You look so depressed. How's Mr. Bananas Foster?"

"I hate Steven" she said with a frown on her face. "I was in love with a creep. I finally went to Steven's apartment. Nothing fancy. He's an auto mechanic.

"He went out to get us a pizza and my insecurities took over. I started checking the closets, the drawers, the bathroom cabinets, and found nothing. I felt stupid for suspecting he was living with a woman.

"Steven came back and we ate our pizza. Then we opened a bottle of wine and he pulled out a guitar and started playing and singing to me. I was slowly melting away. Then he said, 'Dawn, I've never loved anyone this way. I want to take care of you and have a hundred kids.' I said, 'Yes, but I want to wait a year.'

"We made love all night and all the next day too. He told me I was his and his alone, and he was going to buy me a ring

"A couple of days later, my aunt had a party. We're very close, like sisters, and I always tell her everything. Steven and I went to the party and everyone was drinking and eating nonstop. My uncle said to me, 'Come on, Dawn, I have the ping pong table set up. It's my turn to finally win.'

"'Let the competition begin!' Uncle Jim was always a sore loser, but I played him anyway. I was really good and beat him, along with the next five players. Then Steven said with a smile, 'Now it's your turn to lose, Dawn.' Everyone was watching and cheering us on. I played tough and played to win. Steven was superb, but I beat him. I guess he must have gotten embarrassed because he said in a really huffy voice, 'Lets go now!'

"I said goodbye to everyone and as the car pulled away from the house, Steven started screaming at me. 'Who the hell do you think you are, bitch? You're no different than all the other pigs.' Then he smacked me right across the face.

Lucille Fordin

I stopped cutting Dawn's hair. I could fill my blood rushing to my head, "That son of a bitch."

"I was screaming and crying and said, 'Let me out of this car right now. I hate you.' Steven grabbed me and started shaking me and telling me how sorry he was, and that it would never happen again. I cried all night.

"Lucy, my parents never put a hand on me and I wasn't going to let anyone else hit me. I loved Steven so much and I felt in a way that I couldn't live without him, so I gave him another chance."

"Oh, no, Dawn, you didn't."

"He promised he'd never do it again, and I felt I had to believe him. I wanted to believe him. He gave me an engagement ring and now I'm really happy."

"Dawn, promise me if he ever hits you again, walk away. Or should I say, run fast. I had a similar experience when I was twenty-one and I found out that men who hit women don't stop. Please be on your guard."

"Okay, Lucy, I'll be careful and I'll see you in a few months for my highlights."

About six months later Dawn came in the salon and told me the rest of her nightmare.

Once a month she would spend a weekend at his apartment. She asked Steven why he was wasting money in motels when they could be going to his place. He told her he wanted to keep everything exciting for her and that his friends were always in and out of his apartment with their girlfriends. She believed him. Then one day the phone rang in Steven's apartment and when she answered it, the caller hung up on her.

Steven screamed at her, "I told you not to answer the phone, ever! I'm not talking to my father and it probably was him." Just that fast Steven became sweet and loving again and said, "Lets set a date for the wedding. I've waited long enough." So they set a date and just as fast, she forgot about the incident.

She was happy again until one day she received a phone call from a woman named Trish, who claimed to be Steven's wife. She wanted to meet Dawn, but she had just given birth and said she couldn't drive yet. So that meant Dawn would have to go to her.

Dawn screamed into the phone, "You can't be his wife. I was in his apartment and there were no signs of a wife or a baby. We have been together every day for almost a year, and we're engaged to be married in six months. You're crazy, lady, and you're a liar."

"Dawn, I'll prove it to you. Please come while Steven is at work."

Dawn thought about it and made arrangements to meet Trish at her apartment

Dawn knocked on the door and a tall, dark-haired Italian girl greeted her with a baby in her arms. "I'm Trish. Come on in."

"Trish put the baby down for a nap and we proceeded to talk," Dawn said. "She had bruises and marks all over her face and arms. I couldn't believe what I was seeing and hearing.

"'When Steven was growing up, his father would beat him and lock him in the closet overnight because of his uncontrollable temper,' Trish said. "His parents were going to a marriage counselor constantly because of Steven's violent behavior.

"'Trish why do you stay with him if he beats you all the time?'

"'I love him; you know how sweet he can be. Did he play his guitar for you, too? But now I'm afraid of losing him to you. You're not the first girlfriend he's had. We've been married eight years. Once a month I spend a weekend at my mother's; she's very sick. I knew Steven needed some private time alone, but the beatings are getting worse. Steven has told me he would kill the baby if I ever tried to leave him.'

"I swore to Trish I never knew he was married. I don't date married men. I could never be responsible for hurting another woman. I tried to convince Trish that Steven should know that we know his little secret. I knew Steven would never lay another hand on me. Ha, what a joke that was!"

"We decided to wait together in the apartment for him to come home from work so Trish and the baby would be safe. As we talked more, she told me that Steven had told her he had a part-time job at night and on the weekends. He would blame the beatings on her because he had too much pressure working all day and night.

"'Steven never wanted kids,' Trish said. "He tried to beat the baby out of me. One weekend, when I was in the hospital trying to save my

Lucille Fordin

baby, I called our apartment and you answered the phone. I just hung up and went to be with my baby.'

"Lucy, this man would actually pack all Trish's clothes in boxes before I got to his apartment. Then he'd unpack everything when Trish was due home. A real Jekyll and Hyde! I still thought I could change him and he would love me and never beat me. But what a crock of shit that was!

"The door opened and Steven walked in and stared at the two of us for about five minutes. No one said a word. We just stared at each other and then I finally said, 'I guess you have to make a choice now.'

"Steven said nothing, turned around and left. He slammed the door behind him. Trish said, 'I'm dead tonight when he comes back.'

"'Trish, why would you take a chance? I'm through with Steven. Let me take you and the baby to your mother's so you'll be safe. I could never trust him again, Trish. How could you?' Trish refused to leave.

"I left and starting driving home, and before I knew it Steven was behind me blinking his lights and blowing his horn for me to pull over. I was scared to death, and so I stopped the car.

"'Open your door, Dawn.'

"'No way.'

"'Dawn, I love you. I won't hurt you. Please let me explain. I want to marry you. I was leaving Trish when she decided on her own to get pregnant. I didn't know what to do. Please, I love you.'

"Steven started crying and dropped to his knees right there. I opened my car door. He was crying and holding me tight as he explained himself, and it all made sense to me because I wanted to believe him so badly. Then Steven made love to me in the car like he never did before. I gave him another chance. I was sure he loved me and would get a divorce.

"What I didn't know until later was that when Steven went home that night, he made love to Trish, too. He told her he'd leave me and if she ever did something like that again he'd kill her and the baby and no one would ever know who did it.

"That weekend Steven told me they split up for good because he told her he loved me. Then he took me to Disney World for the weekend.

"The following weekend we were out dancing in a club and Dean, a guy I knew from bartending, said 'Hi' and I introduced him to Steven. On the way home, Steven said to me, 'I saw how you looked at Dean, you bitch.' Then he spat in my face and said, 'I'm sure you fucked him, you whore.' He was screaming at me all the way home. I was scared to death. I figured he was just jealous because he loved me, so I forgot all about it. Big mistake!

"One night, he flipped out and grabbed me by the throat and started choking me. When he called me the next day I told him I didn't want to see him anymore. He went crazy and said, 'I'll kill you first before I let you ever leave me.'

"The next weekend I went out with a group of my friends. Steven showed up at the club. I didn't realize he had been following me all week. He was as sweet as sugar that night and convinced me to go outside with him. There were people everywhere so I knew I'd be safe. Steven reassured me he'd get help and would never abuse me again. Then he kissed me. Damn it, Lucy, I felt those tingles all over my body again. I was hooked again. What I didn't know at the time was that Trish had moved back in. You see, when he didn't have Trish to take out his anger on, he took it out on me. Trish and I were being used and we were both too blind to see it . . . or maybe too hooked on his sugar.

"The next day at work the man who parks my car told me that a blond guy was asking questions and stalking me. I told him not to worry, that it was just my jealous boyfriend. One day my car wouldn't start. The next day my tire was flat, and Steven would always appear to save me. How convenient! One night we had an argument and Steven flipped his lid and sucker-punched me right in the face. That was the finishing touch, so to speak. I knew then I was really finished with him.No matter how bad the pain of loving him was, I didn't want him near me anymore. My dreams were finally over. But that's not the end of the story, Lucy."

Uh-oh! My body started trembling, and I felt like I was going to collapse. My face was wrinkled and red from feeling her pain. "Let me sit down," I said. "I can't believe this. Finish this nightmare."

"I came out of work around 2 am. My car wouldn't start. A girl was raped two weeks earlier in the garage. I was scared and no one was around. I had paid off some money I owed to a fellow bartender so I didn't have extra money with me, and I had left my charge card at home. I didn't know what I was going to do. As I started walking away, Steven

Lucille Fordin

pulled up and said, 'Dawn, you can't walk two miles. Please let me drive you home so nothing happens to you. I could never forgive myself. I promise I won't even talk to you if you don't want me to.'

"I hesitated. I was scared of Steven, but more scared of the creeps in the streets late at night. By now the club was closed and everyone was gone, so I felt I had no choice but to take a chance.

"'Steven, do you promise to take me home?'

"'Yes Dawn, I still love you and I promise I won't hurt you.' He was so sincere. I got into the car. Lucy, I am so stupid. Steven drove straight to his apartment.

"'Steven, let me call my girlfriend. She's spending the weekend at my place. She'll definitely be worried, especially when I told her I would be straight home.' I just wanted someone to know where I was. As I was dialing the number, Steven kept saying, 'Dawn, I love you. I just want to talk to you and then I'll take you home.'

"I told my girlfriend where I was and that Steven would bring me home soon. I noticed there were no signs of Trish or the baby. As Steven was begging me to make love to him, the phone rang. It was Trish, and she left this message on the answering machine: 'Steven, I've been calling you all night. Honey, the baby has a fever and we're on our way to the hospital. We'll meet you there. I love you. We'll take the baby home instead of us going back to my mom's.'

"I said, 'Steven, take me home and for God's sake go get your wife and kid. I can see nothing has changed here.' Bad move, bad move. He went berserk.

"'You're not leaving until we talk and make love. I won't let you leave mad. I'll kill Trish for upsetting you."

Steven grabbed me and threw me on the bed and started to force himself on me and in me. I said no and tried to push him off. I got loose and started running for the door. I couldn't believe that, with all the screaming for help I was doing, no one called the police or came to help. I guess the neighbors were used to hearing a lot of fighting. I finally convinced Steven I was calm and I had to use the bathroom. It was like convincing a nasty barking dog to let you pass. The windows in the bedroom were nailed shut so there was no way out of there. I thought if I could get the window open I could scream for help.

Finally Steven opened the door and led me into the bathroom, but he stood by the door so I had no chance to do anything. He pushed me back into the bedroom and started begging me to listen to him. I said to myself, 'Stay calm and maybe if I let him make love to me, then I'll get away safe while he's snoring.' But Steven wasn't acting normal. One minute he was calm and the next minute he was in a rage. I said to Steven, 'Calm down now. I love you and want you to make love to me now.' He smiled, but in a split second said, 'You lying bitch, don't try to humor me,' and he smacked me in the face. 'I'll make love to you when I'm good and God-damn ready.'

"I started screaming and crying. Steven put a knife to my throat and said, 'Shut up now or I'll kill you.' I shut up real fast and listened to every word he had to say. Then he started making love to me, if that's what you want to call it. I acted like I loved it. My mother always told me if I ever get in this kind of trouble, just spread my legs and chances are I'll get out alive.

"I should have been given an Academy Award. I convinced him I still loved him and would marry him. After he was done he took me home. I was black and blue and scared to death. I immediately got a restraining order and threatened Steven that I'd put him in jail if he ever got near me again.

"Later that week I heard Trish went home to Steven. Someone beat Steven up and broke his arms. I think Trish's family had it done. Now the two of them are in counseling.

"Lucy, I'm still looking over my shoulder. I hate men; they're all the same. It'll be a long time before I trust anyone enough to start dating again."

"Dawn you had a horrifying experience. It's one of the worst stories I've heard yet."

Dawn said, "I keep a baseball bat in my car. I'm afraid of guns. One thing I learned was that no woman is strong enough to protect herself against any man — particularly when she's hooked on his sugar!"

"Dawn, I'm so sorry. Time heals all wounds." We hugged, "I know you will never forget this horrible experience, because I never forgot a bad situation I was in. It only made me more careful about choosing men."

Chapter Eleven:
Hot Fudge for a Hot Potato

Clients were coming into the salon asking what the horrible smell was outside the door. The stink started coming in the salon and everyone was getting nauseated, so I went outside to investigate. After sniffing around, I realized the smell was coming from the dirt in the planters lined up in front of my salon.

I called maintenance to report the strange odor. They arrived and determined that someone had put horse manure in the dirt. I decided to save a can of it for further use.

It had to be the little shrimp Pepe. I had heard from clients that Pepe was a big gambler at the racetrack. I knew now that I had to win the war. I would put him out of business if it was the last thing I did. I would show him what a woman in business could do. Competition was a good thing.

Over the next six months a lot of people got sick of Pepe's arrogant attitude and became good clients at my salon.

People say women are the biggest yentas in the world, but I find men gossip just as much and sometimes tell me more than I wish to hear.

Harry is a suave, sixty-five year old widower, tall and thin, with a full head of hair. He's very handsome, retired, and loves to gamble. Every two weeks Harry comes in to Renaldo for a trim.

I was working in the chair next to Renaldo one day when I heard Harry say to Renaldo, "Living in a condo and being a widower is like having my pick of the litter, boy. I can have sex whenever I want it, and I never have to cook. Every night since Estelle passed away, someone is knocking on my door with chicken soup, cookies, cakes, pasta dishes, grilled fish, grilled steaks, stuffed peppers, stuffed chicken . . . you get the picture."

Lucille Fordin

Renaldo burst out laughing, "So has your chicken been stuffed lately?"

I stopped blowing my client's hair because her head was veering off to the left toward Renaldo's chair, and I could barely reach her. She turned her hearing aid up so she could hear better. Now we were both eavesdropping.

"Yes, I've been plucked and stuffed more times than I'd like to remember. I'm making up for the ten years Estelle was sick, may God rest her soul." Harry pointed to his penis and said, "I thought the old boy was dead, but he's more alive than ever. I know I'll never need Viagra."

He chuckled, "Women leave me notes on my car, on my door, on my golf clubs on the course with their phone numbers and an invitation for dinner and sex, usually lots of both. Look at this note, Renaldo. It was on my car this morning."

Renaldo read the note aloud:
>*Dear Harry, please join me for dinner*
>*Friday night. I'll have a limo pick you*
>*up in the lobby at 8pm. The driver will*
>*bring you right to me. I'm fifty-two years*
>*old and I have long red hair. I'm very hot*
>*for you. Hopefully, I've sparked your*
>*interest. I promise I'll be gentle and I'm*
>*sure you'll know me when you see me.*
>   *Love and kisses, Your Secret Admirer.*

"Are you going?" asked Renaldo.

"I'm not sure yet."

"Harry, you can always leave. If it's a fatal attraction, run like hell and don't look back."

Renaldo and Harry laughed so hard I laughed out loud. "I'm sorry, guys. I didn't mean to listen in, but I couldn't help it."

"Lucy, what do you think I should do?"

"Well Harry, do you have any idea who this might be? Is it someone in your building? It might be a friend or relative of someone living there, or they wouldn't have access to your car."

"Lucy, half of the building is either blondes or redheads, and nine out of ten are married," Harry said with a smirk. "I feel like I have a sign on my back reading, It's alive and kicking, girls.

"Make an appointment for me two weeks from today, and if I'm still alive, I'll tell you what happened."

The following day I heard two women who live in Harry's building talking in the salon while they were getting manicures.

"Paula, I saw Harry Fox coming out of apartment 412 last night. I don't know who lives there, do you?"

"No Jean, I don't. Whoever it is just moved in two months ago, but I'm sure she doesn't realize Harry is practically servicing our whole building. I heard half of the women are cooking for him. I always see notes on his door. All the years he lived here, I never saw him cheat on his wife. But since she's passed on, the monster's been let out of the cage. Estelle must be turning over in her grave."

"Paula, he has the perfect name and a perfect body. What a fox he is. I'd do him myself if I had the nerve. Of course, if I got caught, I'd be dead, but oh Sweet Jesus, what a way to go!"

Paula and Jean were laughing like two high school kids. Living in a condo must be like living in a college dorm. Everyone knows everyone's business. There are definitely no secrets in condos.

Over the next two weeks it seemed like everyone was talking about how hot Harry was. I heard women asking Rosie, "When does Harry Fox come in for a haircut? I want an appointment at the same time."

Harry had become the stud flavor of the month. Paula and Jean were acting like vultures. Some Harry-admirers forgot they were even married and had grown children. Nothing seemed to matter to these women other than scoring with Harry! I admit I couldn't wait until Harry came in to the salon to find out what happened on his blind date. I felt as if I were one of the yentas waiting to hear the gossip.

Friday morning finally came. I was glad because Harry was coming in early. I waited patiently until Renaldo was finished cutting Harry's hair and they started talking to each other. The minute he was done, I dropped what I was doing and said to Harry, "Okay, I can't wait another minute. How was your blind date?" Harry and Renaldo burst out laughing.

Lucille Fordin

"Harry, you have to tell Lucy about your life of ecstasy, and don't leave anything out . . . especially about the strawberries and whipped cream." Renaldo and Harry became hysterical, laughing all over again.

"Harry, tell me already."

"Okay, Lucy, here's how it went. Friday night I was in the lobby at eight as directed by my Secret Admirer. I was very excited, but I have to tell you I was a little nervous not knowing what or whom to expect.

"A limo pulled up and the driver said to me, 'You must be Harry Fox.'

"'Yes, I am.'

"'Follow me, sir.'

"I stepped into the car and said to the driver, 'Where are you taking me so I can decide if I still want to go or not?'

"'Sir, I've been given instructions to take you to the Fontainebleu Hotel. I have a key in this envelope with a note for you. No matter how long your business takes you, I'll be waiting to take you home.'

"The note said,

> Dear Harry, I'm glad you decided to meet with me. You won't be sorry. I've ordered an elegant dinner for two, and if you don't like what you see, you may leave after dinner. Please don't change your mind.
>
> Your Secret Admirer.

"I told the driver to proceed. The closer we got to the hotel, the more excited I could feel myself getting. Finally the waiting was over. We were there. As I was going up the elevator I couldn't help but think, 'Boy I hope there's not anybody there waiting to kill me!' I couldn't get my hand to put the key in the door, I was so nervous. I stood there for a moment and said to myself, 'Harry you're being stupid. No one wants to kill you. Put the key in the damn door.' I opened the door and there stood this tall, gorgeous redhead in a skin-tight black, slinky dress.

"'Come on in, Harry.'

I was in shock. There stood Ginger, a beautiful married woman who lived in the penthouse above me.

"'Ginger, it can't be you! What about your husband?'

"'He's away on business and I'm sure he took his girlfriend with him. I haven't slept with Fernando for two years, ever since I found out about his affairs.'

"'Ginger, you're a beautiful woman. Why do you stay with him and waste your life?'

" 'Fernando won't give me a divorce, so I decided to stay with him and do to him what he's been doing to me. I might as well be 'miserable rich,' than 'miserable poor.'"

Ginger made her way over to my side of the room, and practically touching me with her breasts, she said, 'Harry, please stay and have dinner with me and let's forget about Fernando. Dinner is on its way up. Will you dine with me? If you feel you don't want to stay, I won't stop you from leaving. But darling, if I were you, I wouldn't miss dessert. I can guarantee you'll never forget it.'

"'May I ask who or what is for dessert?'

"With a sexy chuckle Ginger said, 'You'll have to wait and find out,' as she pressed her lips gently on mine. I knew there and then I was putty in her hands, as the blood rushed through my body.

"We talked all through dinner. Somehow I forgot Ginger was married and lived in the penthouse a few floors above me. I tried to convince myself Fernando was a creep and didn't deserve Ginger—a sweet, beautiful, sexy redhead with piercing blue eyes who had me totally mesmerized within an hour. Lucy, are you sure you want to hear this?"

"Harry, if you stop now, I'll shave your head bald!"

"Okay Lucy, here it goes. We had just opened our second bottle of champagne when Ginger leaned over and said, 'Harry, dessert will be here shortly. Will you stay?'

"Ginger slowly moved in very close to me and pressed her body to mine. I could feel my heart pounding along with every other part of my body as I heard myself blurt out, 'Yes I'll stay. Of course! I wouldn't miss this for the world.' Ginger leaned in and pressed her lips on mine. Then she said, 'Harry, I'm going to freshen up.'

"Just then there was a knock at the door and a voice said, 'Room Service.' I was relieved and opened the door. Ginger was still in the powder room and I couldn't wait any longer so I had to sneak a peek at the

Lucille Fordin

dessert. The entire table was full. It looked like there was enough to feed the Miami Dolphins.

"I slowly lifted each lid. I found strawberries, hot fudge, whipped cream, and everything else you can think of to make a super sundae, except they forgot the ice cream. I quickly put the lids back as I heard the powder room door open. Ginger came out in a turquoise negligee. Lucy, I'm not exaggerating, she looked like something right out of Playboy. She was simply divine. I knew I was dead meat!

"Ginger said with a smile on her face, 'Harry, this is all for you and you only.'

"'Ginger, I feel I'm a very lucky man to be in the presence of such a beautiful woman.' I walked over to her and started kissing her passionately. As I went to pull away I said, 'Dessert has arrived. Would you like some or would you like to wait till later?'

"'Harry, let me see if they sent everything I ordered.' Ginger opened each tray as she licked her lips and said, 'I love hot fudge, don't you? Harry, I hope you're ready for all of this.'

"'But Ginger, they forgot the ice cream.'

"'We don't need ice cream. You're gonna be my ice cream, Harry.'

"I could have melted the hot fudge if I were near it. I hoped I wouldn't drop dead from a heart attack. Ginger slowly started undressing me. As she put a strawberry dipped in whipped cream in my mouth, she proceeded to lick the excess off of my lips. Every inch of my body was on fire with passion. The hot fudge cooled off, but was still warm when Ginger poured it slowly from my mouth, down my neck, from nipple to nipple, down my stomach, into my bellybutton, around my testicles and on my penis. Just talking about it gets me excited. I hope I'm not offending you, Lucy."

"Don't stop Harry. I need to learn some new tricks. What happened next?"

"Ginger put a cherry in my bellybutton and two rings of pineapple around my nipples. She dropped nuts slowly on my penis and it rose for the occasion."

Just listening to Harry talk gave me tingles. His deep voice was so sexy. My receptionist Rosie called me to the phone. "Take a message, Rosie. I'm very busy."

The salon could have burned down but I wasn't about to miss the rest of Harry's story. "What happened next, Harry?"

"Ginger started licking everything off. It was glorious. We were both a mess, so we took a hot shower. As we slowly washed each other, I felt like a teenager. We had sex on the bedroom floor, soaking wet. One hour later, we made love in bed in a slow, gentle, traditional way. I was limping when I left the room."

We chuckled and I told Harry not to stop.

"Lucy, I had a night like I've never had in my life. Estelle was sick for so long, but I stayed loyal to her. I feel a little guilty now, but I shouldn't because Estelle has been gone for a long time. Ginger took me by surprise, but I just couldn't stop myself. Once I cooled off, I knew that I could never see Ginger again unless she got a divorce."

"Harry, be careful," I said. Women can be worse than men sometimes, especially if they're in heat. Just remember that a hard pecker has no conscience and it could definitely get you in trouble."

"Lucy, I never knew it was so easy getting what you want. I had a good clean woman all my life. I better slow down now that I've had a taste of single life. I wonder if I'll ever find someone like Estelle?"

"Oh yes, you will, but I think you should be a little more careful of what you do with the women living in your building. I've heard you've had half of the women there, you hot potato."

"Lucy, I feel so embarrassed. I was like a little kid in a candy store . . . make that soda shop. I'm going to think about selling my apartment and starting a new life. Thanks for telling me. I thought no one knew anything. I'll see you again in two weeks. I'll tell you what I decide to do."

Two weeks later, Harry came into the salon for an appointment. Renaldo was running late, and I had just finished a client. I couldn't wait to talk to Harry. "Harry, can I get you some coffee? I'll join you while you're waiting."

"Lucy, I decided to wait a few months before putting my apartment up for sale. Ginger sent me another note, but I decided not to meet her. She's married, and it can only lead to trouble. I'll never forget the evening I spent with her. I still get a rush every time I see her. Then I remember she's married, and I cool off quickly. I was out of control, and I'm going to take a break from dating."

Lucille Fordin

I didn't hear much gossip about Harry in the months to come. A year later Harry sold his apartment and moved to Fisher Island. He met a lovely woman, got married, and is very happy to this day.

Chapter Twelve:
Have the Lizards and Frogs Stood Up and Applauded You Yet?

Truck drivers have very active lives. I've been cutting Leo's hair for eight years. He's told me some crazy stories but this one, takes the cake.

Leo drove a truck back and forth from Pittsburgh to Miami, delivering paper goods. A man of fifty-two, he never thought much of dating. He dedicated his life to being mother and father to his two children after his wife passed away from breast cancer in 1992. His daughter is eighteen and his son twenty-two. Both children still live at home.

The minute Leo told me he was from Pittsburgh, we became friends. One day in August, Leo came in for his haircut and told me he was in love with a forty-year-old woman named Angela. He met her at a local bar near his hotel in Miami. While I was cutting his hair, I asked Leo how his life was going.

"Lucy, I've been dating Angela for six months and I'm simply in love."

"Leo, I'm so happy for you. Tell me about Angela."

"Angela has two kids, ten and twelve. She's a waitress at O'Hara's Bar and Grill. I go there every time I'm in Miami. I've been looking at her for a year, but I just couldn't get up the nerve to ask her out. I assumed she was married, since all she ever talked about was her two kids.

"One night Angela walked over to me and said, 'Leo, I'll be done working at 2:00 am. Would you like to take me out for breakfast?' Without any hesitation I said, 'Yes!'

Lucille Fordin

"Lucy, it was like we connected immediately. She told me she had been separated for six months and was waiting for her divorce to be final. She rented a room to a college girl who baby-sat her kids. It worked out well for both of them. She's a dedicated mother. Tonight I'm going to Angela's for dinner, and I'll finally get to meet her children.

"Leo, I'm very happy for you, but can I ask you a personal question?"

"Yes, Lucy."

"How come in six months she's never invited you to her house?"

"Because Angela always felt that unless we were serious, she didn't want to cause any more trauma to her children, since their father left home."

"That makes sense to me. If you want to make friends with the kids, just take a lot of candy with you. It works for me with my nephews. If not, try money." We both laughed and I wished him good luck.

The next time I saw him, Leo said he was going to propose to Angela.

"I guess she got the divorce, huh?" I said. Leo hesitated, a strange look on his face. "Not quite. Her husband is trying to take the kids from her. The divorce should be final next month. Lucy, I love Angela so much. She's so honest and unassuming, plus she's a good cook. You know how I love to eat. Some nights after she finishes work, instead of going to my hotel, we go back to her house. The kids are sleeping so we lie out on the patio looking up at the stars for hours, talking."

"Leo, are you sure you're just 'talking' under that romantic Miami moon? Have the lizards and frogs stood up and applauded you yet?"

"Lucy, you're crazy. What a sense of humor you have."

Angela accepted the ring but wanted to wait a year before she moved back to Pittsburgh with Leo. She told him it would be hard to take the kids away from their father and friends. Her husband threatened to kill her if she ever moved the kids away.

The next time I saw Leo, he had a long face.

"Hi, Lucy. I broke up with Angela and I'm very depressed."

"Leo, what happened?"

"I found out she was a liar and a cheater. She had me fooled! Do you have time for me to tell you what happened?"

I was dying to know. In a sympathetic voice I said, "I always have time for you, Leo. Please go on."

"A couple of months ago I was driving to Miami and stopped in Jacksonville to get something to eat. Sitting next to me were two truckers talking loudly.

"One said to the other, 'I can't wait to see the look on my wife's face when I get home early. I'm not due home for two weeks. I think the bitch is having an affair. I plan on castrating whoever it is. My kids told me, "Mommy's friend from work is a nice guy. He brings us candy and presents." The bitch had him in my house, and if I ever find out it's true, I'll throw her out and she'll never see the kids again. Then when I get done with her, I'm going to find out who he is, and he'll be sorry he ever laid a hand on my wife, I can tell you that. I work day and night. I don't like being away from home two weeks at a time, but hey, it pays the bills. Let's go, man. I want to be there when she gets done with work so I can follow her. And God help her if she's not alone!'

"Lucy, you were right about the candy and presents. The kids loved them. I couldn't help thinking all the way to Miami that the story I heard sounded so like my situation, but I knew it couldn't be, so I forgot about it. I was sure it was just a coincidence and I was only being paranoid.

"That night after work, Angela said to me, 'Leo, let's go back to my house. I'll make us breakfast. The kids aren't feeling well.' Lucy, for some reason I was still feeling uneasy so I told Angela I was tired and that she should be with the kids in case they needed her. She understood and I told her I'd call her the next day.

"I couldn't sleep, so an hour later I decided to drive past her house to see if a truck was there. I figured I was being stupid, but I couldn't help myself. Okay, there was one chance in ten million that his truck would be in front of her house. Lucy, it was a nightmare. All the lights were on in the house. I could hear yelling coming from inside. The truck was there. The next day I got a phone call from Angela.

"'Leo, I have to see you. My husband came here last night and took my kids to his mother's. He knew all about us and beat me up very badly.'

"'Angela, I'll be right over.'

"'No,' she screamed in a panic. 'I'll come to the hotel in a couple of hours.'

Lucille Fordin

"Angela showed up three hours later and proceeded to tell me nothing but lies. I told her what I heard at the truck stop and told her we were finished. I never wanted to see her again. How could she do this to me? All the lies she fed me and the secrets she had."

"Leo, maybe you should give her a chance. After all, she is divorced, isn't she?"

"No, she lied about that, too. It took me a couple of hours of listening to her until I said, 'Just tell me the truth.'

"'Leo I'm sorry. I never meant to hurt you, but I was so lonely. I didn't plan on falling in love with you. Yes, I'm married, but I'll leave him, I promise.'

"Lucy, Angela's husband is also a trucker. When I was in Miami, he was in New York. Angela and I made love in his bed. I ate his food. I spent time with his children. What kind of woman is she? How could she do this to me or anyone else? She used me and, as far as I'm concerned, she's a whore! I could never trust her again, no matter what. My dear wife was a virgin when I married her. She's dead now, but the whores live on. I really don't want anything to do with women if this is how they are."

"Leo, I'm sorry you caught a bad one, but there's a lot of good women out there. You can't let one bad apple stop you from enjoying the rest of your life. You're a good person and you'll find the right woman someday."

Leo didn't date for a year. Finally he liked another woman and found out within a few months that she was an alcoholic.

The next woman made a spectacle out of herself in the middle of dinner at a restaurant. "She put her hand between my legs and grabbed my penis."

That ended his dating. Leo thinks all women are whores, and three years later he's still alone. He refuses to go out with anyone. Angela tried to contact Leo for about a year, but he would never return her phone calls or answer her letters. Another good man ruined for life because of a few stupid, loose women, while the good women sit home and watch TV. I don't know what you want to call it. Bad luck? A bad choice of women ruined Leo's faith in women forever.

Now when Leo comes into the salon, he tells me trucker stories about what he sees on the road. Some are funny, while some are tragic.

Leo was driving down the interstate when he saw a black Chevy in front of him. A pair of bare feet popped out of the right rear side of the car. Within seconds, another pair of feet popped out of the left rear side. As he got closer, two feet appeared on the rear panel. When Leo finally got beside the car, he saw one male and two females in their twenty's stark naked having sex. It looked like a jigsaw puzzle.

It was getting dark. In the distance, he saw a woman near the side of the road. He slowed down and the woman screamed, "Stop the car!"

Leo jammed on his brakes to help the woman. She was around forty-five years old, and was crying and talking so fast Leo didn't know what she was saying. Leo said, "Slow down and tell me what happened. Should I call the police?"

"No, no, no!"

"Do you need an ambulance?"

"No, no, no!"

"Did you have a fight?"

"No!"

"Have you been kidnapped?"

"No!"

"What's your name?"

"Judy."

"I'm Leo. I can't leave you here. Will you tell me what happened?"

Judy was sobbing and could barely talk. "My husband left me here. We had a flat tire, and my husband was pissed off. While he was changing the tire, I went into the bushes to go to the bathroom, and I saw the car pull out."

"Judy, where were you when he pulled the car over?"

"In the back, sleeping. But I told him I'd be right back."

"Judy, he probably thought you got back in the car."

"I don't know." She started crying hysterically again.

"Judy, I can't leave you here. Let me call the police or drive you to the next truck stop. Maybe he'll realize you're not in the car."

Twenty minutes later Judy finally got up and started to get into the truck. A car pulled up, and a man jumped out and said, "I was only gone a few minutes and you picked up a man, you bitch."

Lucille Fordin

Judy started crying, and said, "You left me here to die, you pig. Leo could have raped me."

"Okay, I've had enough," Leo said. "Your wife went to the bathroom in the bushes, and you left her here. I tried to help. I didn't rape anyone. I'm gay. Good-bye and good luck."

Leo got into the truck, talking to himself. "I know I'm not gay, but I don't have any luck with women. Maybe next time Judy will piss in a bucket! In the car."

A few months later, Leo pulled into a rest area in Georgia to get some sleep. He had just dozed off when there was a knock on his window. "Hey, mister, you want some sex, $30.00?"

Leo said, "No, go away."

Five minutes later, "Hey mister, you want a blow job, $25.00?"

Leo said, "No, and don't come back."

Leo noticed a girl arguing with a guy. The girl was around fifteen, and the guy was in his thirties. Leo tried to go back to sleep, but there was another knock at his window.

"Hey, mister, please, I'll do anything you want for $20.00."

Leo said, "No, go away."

The girl kept pounding on his window and said, "Please do something or my father won't let me come home with him."

"That's your father? Your father's a pimp?" Leo was really pissed. He rolled down the window, started the truck, and as he pulled out he screamed at the man, "What kind of father are you? I'm calling the police."

Leo decided to get something to eat, so he pulled into the next rest stop. While he was having coffee and dessert, a woman sat down next to him and said, "Is that pie good?"

"Yes, it's very good." Leo continued eating and ignored the woman.

She was in her forty's and on the heavy side, with stringy brown hair and breasts as big as watermelons. "Do you live around here? My name is Candy. What's yours?"

'My name is Leo, and I'm not interested."

Candy jumped out of her seat and in a loud voice said, "What's the matter? Aren't I good enough for you?"

Leo ignored her. Candy clutched her breast and said in a crazy voice, "Do you know why they call me Candy? Because these are sweet."

Leo went to the register to pay his bill, when he heard, "Hey Leo, where are you going? Don't you want a piece of candy?"

Everyone turned to look at him as he walked out the door, talking to himself. "I really don't have any luck with women. Maybe I should turn gay! Nah, not today."

Chapter Thirteen:
Tarzan Wants To Pump You Up

Hurricane season can be very scary in Florida, especially after hurricane Andrew in 1992. Zane, one of my top hair stylists, lost everything he owned in that brutal storm. I felt lucky I only had forty thousand dollars in damages.

A month later, people in Florida were still trying to get over their fears and put their lives back together again. But every time it rained, people would panic. To this day there are still people who haven't recovered from that hurricane.

A man walked into the salon for a haircut. He looked familiar to me, but I couldn't remember where I knew him from. He said to Rosie, "I need a haircut with whoever you recommend. My barber is on vacation. My name is David Green."

Rosie called me to the front of the salon, "Lucy, Mr. Green wants to know if you have time to cut his hair. I see you're in the middle of placing orders and have no time. Mr. Green, Lucy is the owner and Zane is excellent with men's haircuts. Get your hair washed and he'll do you right away."

As Mr. Green walked away, I asked Rosie what that was all about. "Lucy, he said he wanted the girl with the blonde hair and big boobs."

We laughed. Rosie said, "I had to keep him away from you. I can tell he's a little goofy. Zane can handle him."

Rosie is always very protective of me and I trust her with my life.

"Lucy, he looks familiar to me, but I can't place him. Keep an eye on Romeo. He's flirting with all the women."

Rosie is very pretty, a natural blonde with black roots. Ha! Ha! She's in her mid-sixties. She and her husband had a beautiful marriage and worked side by side when they owned a very large hair salon in Miami. Rose's four children protect her and love her like she loves and protects me. I feel the same way about her. She tried to keep her business running after her husband died, but it was too much work and had too many memories. She sold the salon and came to work for me. Rosie is excellent for me and the salon.

Zane moved to Miami from New York. He is one of the most gifted hairdressers I've ever come across. He can look at a face and the way a person dresses, and give them a perfect cut, style or color to enhance their beauty.

He's handsome, has a good heart and a fabulous personality. He's always booked solid and there's always a waiting list for his appointments. He's worked for me for fifteen years, and we're the best of friends. As a favor to me, he squeezed Mr. Green in for a haircut.

As I walked by Zane's chair I heard Mr. Green say, "I'm going to be Tarzan after tomorrow. I'm having a pump put in."

Zane looked at me and rolled his eyes in a way that made it difficult for me to hold back my laughter. Zane said, "I'm sorry your swimming pool pump was destroyed in the hurricane."

Mr. Green looked puzzled. "Pool pump? My pool is fine. I'm talking about a penis pump. Do you think Lucy will let me try it out on her, or how about that sexy Spanish hairdresser over there? That Rosie is also sexy."

Zane laughed and said, "Chichi is single. Lucy won't date clients, and Rosie is happily married again to a wonderful guy. You don't want to mess around with Rosie anyway; she'll deflate your pump and twist it around your ears. I'm sure you'll find a lot of women to use your pump on, Mr. Tarzan. It was nice meeting you and good luck tomorrow."

Mr. Green paid his bill and left. Zane was laughing so hard when he told me Mr. Green wanted Rosie and Chichi at the same time. "He wanted to try out his new pump on all of you."

Rosie said, "Maybe we should think about it. We'll let the jerk pump it up, Chichi can hold it, and I'll cut it off for him." There wasn't a dry eye in the salon. We were all laughing hysterically. Have I mentioned how good it is for you to laugh?

Hair Network Secrets Told in a Salon

A month later Mr. Green's wife Jean came in the salon for her hair color. I was doing her color when she said, "Lucy, that hurricane was a disaster for me."

I said, "Me too, Jean. I had forty thousand dollars in damages. How much damage did you have?"

"My home wasn't damaged too badly, but my body would like to leave town on a vacation."

"Your body!"

"Yes, Lucy, I'm exhausted. I'm sixty-four years old and my stupid husband had a cheap roof put on the house and used the rest of the insurance money on a stupid penis pump. I think he's trying to kill me! All day and all night he's pumping his thing up and down. David is seventy years old and he has always been oversexed. I was glad when his penis dropped dead from all of his medications. If he keeps this up he'll be dead from a heart attack by the time he turns seventy-one."

I couldn't believe Jean was married to a jerk like David. If she only knew! In the weeks to come, David became a popular name in the salon.

One day a client named Ethel came in with a broken pelvic bone. She told everyone her boyfriend "David" was making love to her "like an animal" and broke her pelvic bone.

"Ethel, are you all right? I heard what happened. What a lucky woman you are. No one has ever broken my bones in bed before. How did you drive to the salon in all that pain?"

"My boyfriend drove me. He's waiting outside. I want you to meet him."

"Ethel, I'd love to meet the sex machine." Ethel was a lovely lady. It was a shame she didn't know he was married, not to mention sleeping with other women.

I couldn't wait to see the look on Mr. Tarzan Pump-Boy's face when I wheeled Ethel out to the car in her wheel chair. David's eyes opened wide with fear on his face.

"It's nice to meet you, David. I've heard so much about you."

David practically threw Ethel in the car and said, "We're in a hurry to get to the doctor's office. Nice meeting you."

Lucille Fordin

The following day David called me at the salon. "Lucy, it's David Green. I wanted to thank you for not telling on me. How about meeting me for coffee so I can explain."

"You don't have to answer to anyone but your wife. Remember her? I think you have enough women to handle."

Saturday morning Jean came in for her regular appointment. While she was having her hair washed, David came in with two dozen doughnuts. "Hi, Lucy. This is for taking such good care of my beautiful wife." Then he leaned over and kissed me on the lips. Yuck! "Jean, your hairdresser is a beautiful woman. Can we take her home with us?"

I couldn't help but think, "What a creep!" While I was doing Jean's hair, David was telling jokes, trying to prove to me that he was a class act. Every time Jean turned her head away, David would wink at me. Again, Yuck! Him Tarzan, me Sick. He was repulsive. I felt like he was undressing me the whole time.

Over the next few weeks David became a real pain in the ass, running in and out of the salon with cookies and doughnuts. He really thought he was some hot stud. I couldn't tell Jean what was going on. It seemed like the ruder I was to him the more he liked it. It reached the point where I couldn't get him to stay away. Rosie would make up story after story as to why I couldn't take his phone calls. David was being very persistent, I'll give him that.

One day a beautiful arrangement of flowers was delivered to the salon. Rosie's mouth dropped wide open and she got this strange look on her face.

"Oh my God, please don't tell me these beautiful flowers are from that jerk." The note on the flowers read:
> *Dear Lucy, please have dinner with me.*
> *I think you're very beautiful. I can*
> *give you great pleasure. You only live*
> *once!*
>   *Your Secret Admirer.*

Rosie and I looked at each other in amazement. I couldn't believe that David Green was being so persistent, especially after being told "No" at least five times.

"Rosie, the next time he calls, give me the phone. I'll stop the jerk forever."

Two hours later I heard Rosie's voice over the loudspeaker. "Lucy, I have an important call for you."

"Hello, can I help you? This is Lucy."

"Yes, you can. It's your Secret Admirer. Do you like your flowers?"

"Mr. Green, the flowers are beautiful. Thanks for trying again, but the answer is still no! Now listen closely. It will always be no. Do I want to have anything to do with you? No, not now, not ever. Now, which part don't you understand? I WANT NOTHING TO DO WITH YOU. If you don't leave me alone, I'll be forced to tell your wife. I don't want you calling here, and I don't want you running in and out of the salon all day. Now do you understand what no means? If you think I'm kidding, just try me." I slammed the phone down in his ear.

Rosie overheard the conversation and said, "Lucy, I wouldn't have been so nice to him. I hope he doesn't call here anymore because if he does, I'll fix him real good. You know what I think? I think we should go out with him and pump that sucker up until it explodes. Then for sure he won't bother us anymore."

I was taken aback for a second because it wasn't like Rosie to say things like that. We burst out laughing and couldn't stop.

David made it a point to drive his wife back and forth to the salon. I couldn't hurt this sweet, naïve wife, who wouldn't hurt a fly, so we just ignored him.

Saturday afternoon Alma Long came in for her regular appointment. While I was doing her hair, she proceeded to tell me this not-so-surprising story.

"Lucy, I'm in love with a married man. He's so good in bed. He's going to leave his wife. He's in love with me. He told me that his wife has cancer. Look what he did to my hair this morning; it's a mess. He's such an animal. I opened the door and before I knew it he was all over me. David was sucking my ears, kissing my nose, licking my luscious lips when he grabbed my breast and almost knocked me over with his passion. I completely forgot about how bad my back was hurting. That's why I'm limping now. I loved every minute of it. Not too many men his age can have sex. When David looks at me he can't control himself. He

Lucille Fordin

must love me because he tells me, 'Just knowing I'm coming to see you makes me hot. By the time I reach your apartment I have a hard on.'"

"Alma who is this David? Do you know anything about him or his past? Does he have a last name? What does he look like?"

I don't know why I bothered. There was no question in my mind that Alma was also sleeping with Tarzan, along with four other women who were clients in my salon, and I had heard the same stories from them. None of them seemed to care he was married. They all thought he was a good guy for taking care of his sick wife. What a smooth talker.

Six months later, Tarzan slipped from his vine. David Green had a heart attack. I wasn't surprised. Five months later he was back in action with a new group of women.

.

Chapter Fourteen:
I Want My Two Hundred Bucks Back

It was Labor Day weekend. September was a slow month in Florida, so I decided it was time to remodel the salon again. I had remodeled certain areas three times already. I reversed the front desk and makeup station twice. The manicure stations were back to back until I put them in a straight line to give the manicurists more room to move around.

I had one room for facials and waxing until I decided two rooms were better. I planned to get rid of the massage area. I found out it's not good for clients to be able to listen to each other's conversations with only a curtain between them. I don't have enough room to make two enclosed rooms. A massage area for my salon wasn't profitable because it took up so much space.

I was doing battle with my tape measure, trying to decide whether to enlarge the waiting area or make a private lunch area for the employees, when I noticed a handsome man at the front desk. He was wearing all black, and looked like he was in his late forties. He was tall and thin, dressed very elegantly, and had an earring in one ear. His dark hair and dark eyes made him look very European. Actually, he looked like a gloriously handsome pimp. He was talking to, Rosie.

"I want the owner to do my girlfriend's hair." He nodded at a short woman beside him. I heard about this place all the way up in Ft. Lauderdale. That's why we're here."

Over the loudspeaker, I heard, "Lucy, please come to the front desk."

"Rosie, what can I do for you?"

"This gentleman would like you to do his girlfriend's hair. Do you have time?"

Lucille Fordin

"I just had a cancellation so right now would be a good time. My name is Lucy, what's yours?" I asked his girlfriend, a brunette about twenty-seven and nothing special to look at.

"Joan," she replied.

"Joan, please have your hair washed and conditioned. I'll be at my station."

When she returned, I had her sit down in my chair. "Joan, do you know how you would like your hair cut, or are you leaving it up to me?"

"Do what you think is right for me."

I decided to make small talk. "Your husband is a nice man."

"Oh, he's my boyfriend and I love him very much. One day soon I know we'll get married."

I proceeded to give her a haircut and blow. Joan's hair was two inches past her shoulders, long and stringy. I cut it shoulder length, with bangs. "How do you like your hair?"

Joan said, "Lucy, I love it! I'm sure Brad will love it too."

Brad showed no reaction at all when Joan walked over to him smiling. Brad thanked me and said, "We'll see you soon."

A few weeks later Brad came in with another girl named Candy, a pretty blonde around thirty years old. He left the salon and said he would be back in an hour.

Candy also said she was Brad's girlfriend and planned to marry him someday. Neither one of us mentioned Joan. Candy had short hair that made her look like a drowned rat. I decided to layer and spike her hair with gel to give her a punky look, leaving some hair flowing down her long neck.

I found it amazing how different Brad's taste was in women. Brad came back to pick Candy up but didn't say a word.

Candy was smiling and told me she loved her hair. Brad still said nothing. He looked at me with his shifty eyes, like he was flirting, and made me feel very uncomfortable. I said, "Brad, do you like Candy's hair?"

He said, "I like your hair better, Lucy."

Candy's face dropped in disappointment. I told her not to pay any attention to Brad's sarcastic remark. She looked beautiful, I said.

As Brad and Candy turned to leave the salon, he said, "Hey, babe, thanks for cutting my girlfriend's hair. We'll be back."

As I walked back to my station, my employees sounded like a church choir as they mimicked Brad. "Hey, babe." I loved it. We laughed all week. I always wanted to be a "babe."

A week later, I was giving Cleo, one of my regular clients, a perm at the shampoo station. As I was finishing the procedure, I looked up and saw Brad at the front desk with another girl. This one was a redhead, around thirty-five.

I was so busy trying to figure out who this girl was that I dropped Cleo's head in the sink. As her head proceeded to bounce around, I apologized to her and said, "I'm so sorry."

"Lucy, you gave me a headache. Is my head bleeding?

"No."

"Are you trying to kill me? I think I have whiplash."

I had been doing Cleo's hair for five years. She had a great sense of humor, so I was pretty sure that she didn't have whiplash and wasn't planning to sue me. I've never had a lawsuit, and can only hope I never do. When I explained to Cleo why I dropped her head, she said, "Hurry up, drop my head and run up to the front desk. Let me know who the third girl is before you kill me altogether." We laughed.

I walked up to the front desk and said, "Hi, Brad. Who's this beautiful redhead?"

Brad had walked in without making an appointment. "This is Lori. Can you fit her in between your appointments?" She was overweight, at least a size sixteen, and had a pretty face with thick, beautiful red hair. Dyed red hair, of course!

I told Brad I would take care of her. Lori sat in my chair and told me she was Brad's girlfriend and planned on marrying him some day.

I told Lori to get her hair shampooed and I would give her a conditioner on the house. The conditioner is a nice way to keep a client busy while another client is getting finished.

I quickly went to see if Cleo's "whiplash" was better. Cleo was still laughing at me bouncing her head all over the sink and only wanted to know the story. I told her what I knew while I cut her hair, and promised to tell her the rest at her next appointment.

Lucille Fordin

Lori came back to my chair and we discussed how she wanted her hair done. I suggested blonde highlights, done very fine throughout her hair. The haircut was easy, spiked bangs with the hair cut in layers toward her face. It made her chubby, round face look much thinner. I was very proud of my work. Lori looked beautiful. I know what it's like to be overweight. At one time I was 250 pounds. I've been a yoyo with my weight all my life. I'm 150 pounds now, and my need to please a heavy person is very important to me.

"Lori, how do you like your hair?"

"Lucy, it's never been so beautiful. I love my hair and I hope Brad likes it too."

Brad showed up at the salon and never said a word to Lori. "Lucy," he said to me, "if you ever sell this place and need a job, give me a call. Here's my card. You could make a lot of money working for me."

I looked at the card but didn't understand what it meant. It said, "Brad is the man who can deliver. "Salesman of the year," and a phone number.

"Brad, what kind of salesman are you?" I could have swallowed my tongue. Lori's face dropped to the floor. I could tell she was pissed off at Brad, but she never said a word.

Brad said, "Call me, Lucy, and I'll show you what kind of salesman I am. Thanks, babe, for everything."

I felt as if I had been struck by lightning. Book smart I'm not, street smart I am. Brad had to be a pimp.

Two days later Brad showed up at the salon with all three girls! He said with a mean, forceful voice to Rosie, "Your boss ruined my girls' hair. I want my two hundred dollars back, plus three hundred for me having to take them somewhere else to get their hair done again. Look at them. They're a mess. I couldn't sell them if I wanted too."

The three girls looked like their heads were dunked in a bucket of water and hung out to dry. Rosie called me to the front desk. I spotted Brad and his girls and as I got closer to the desk, I heard Brad say, "I don't want to look at her face now. Just give me my money back, you bitch."

As I approached the front desk, I said, "Watch your mouth, Brad. What did you do to these girls? I wasn't born yesterday."

Brad was nasty and getting more aggressive as he turned toward me. He was practically on top of me. I could smell his nasty breath while spit flew out of his mouth onto my face as he cursed me.

I had enough of Brad's mouth. The clients started moving toward the back of the salon and the hairdressers followed, trying to keep the clients calm. I heard Zane say, "Don't worry about Lucy. She'll fix that creep. I'm ready for a good fight. I better go help."

Zane never got a chance to make it to the front desk. The street girl in me reacted fast while Rosie threatened to call the police. I looked up at this 6'2" giant and said, "Go pull your con somewhere else, mister. I won't give you a penny back. Now if you want to call the police or get a lawyer, just remember that this will be the last con job you ever pull, you asshole. Get the fuck out."

Well, I have to tell you I sounded like a truck driver. I even scared myself a little. Rosie's eyes were open super-wide as she just gawked at me. I didn't know I had it in me until it was all over and I began to shake. I didn't stop shaking for two days. I must have been convincing, because Brad left with the girls and I never saw him again, thank God.

I called our mall security guard and told him what happened. I also told him that I followed them to their car to get a license plate number. For two weeks after that incident, all the stores were complaining about being robbed while a man and three girls were in their store. I told Security that Brad threatened me. "Please, could you keep an extra eye out on the salon for the time being?"

Two days later I was told that Brad and his girls got busted trying to rob one of the stores. The security office wouldn't tell me which store was robbed, only that they caught them with the merchandise in their pockets. They ended up going to jail. The police said they had been trying to catch them for three years, and thanks to my description and information, their quest was over.

Chapter Fifteen:
Jill, the Blonde, and the Pill

Mr. Solo was a sweet, trustworthy man. He was married to the same woman for forty years. One day his wife asked him for a divorce. He was devastated. She was in love with Mr. Solo's business partner. For ten years she had been having an affair and no one had a clue what was going on until they both got divorces and went to California together.

Mr. Solo was in Jessie's chair getting a manicure. Jessie has worked for me for ten years. She is Jewish, lots of fun and very busy all the time.

Jill was in Mila's chair getting a manicure. Mila is Russian and has worked for me for five years. She's a perfect lady and never gets involved personally with the clients. A very good trait.

Mr. Solo was getting a manicure when Jill looked at him and said, "My name is Jill. I think you know my husband, Larry Falk. He passed away two years ago."

"The name doesn't ring a bell, but I'm sure he had to be a great guy." Jill asked if he was married. "No, I'm divorced."

I was applying a color in the dye area when I heard Jill speaking to Mr. Solo. I worked slowly so I could hear their conversation.

Jill said, "In that case, how would you like to come to a party I'm having at the country club? I'm celebrating my 50th birthday. There will be over a hundred people at the club tonight. If I didn't invite a good-looking man like you to meet all the single women going to be there, they'd kill me. I promise you'll have a great time." Jill had a sparkle in her eyes and was blushing. I could tell she was interested in Mr. Solo and he looked pretty taken by her.

Lucille Fordin

Jessie couldn't wait for a chance to get into the conversation. I heard her say, "Mr. Solo, if you don't want to go alone to the party, take me. My husband is out of town."

I finished putting the color on and decided to break up Jessie's conversation. She thought she was being cute while Jill thought Jessie was being rude. I heard her tell Mila, "Jessie has some nerve interrupting me."

Mila said, "Don't be upset, Jill. Jessie probably thought she was helping. Your nails and hair look beautiful. You're ready for a great party."

Jill smiled and, as she passed Mr. Solo, she said in a sweet voice, "Please be my guest this evening, Mr. Solo. You'll have a great time. Do you have a first name?"

Mr. Solo smiled at Jill and said, "John, and I'll do my best to show up tonight. Thanks for inviting me."

"Mr. Solo, I couldn't help but overhear your conversation with Jill. She's a lovely lady. It's time you got off your duff and go out."

"Maybe you're right, Lucy. I liked Jill and I think I'll go tonight."

Mr. Solo showed up at the party with a dozen roses in his hand. Jill came running toward him when he entered and said, "You made it. The flowers are beautiful, but you didn't have to bring anything."

"Pretty flowers for a pretty lady. Save a dance for me later. I know you're busy now greeting your guests."

"John, let me introduce you to some people and then I'll see you later."

Jill made her introductions. John went to the bar, sat down and had a drink. Before he knew it, a young woman had started talking to him. "What's your name?"

"John Solo," he replied.

"John, are you family or a friend of Jill's?"

"A new friend, I hope, and you?"

"My name is Lynn. I don't really know Jill. I'm here with my boyfriend, but I'm breaking up with him. He has a bad temper, especially when he drinks. I always end up taking a cab home. But I wanted to come to this party. I was sure I'd meet a nice-looking guy like you. You'll give me a ride home if I need it, won't you?"

"When the time comes and I'm ready to go, Lynn, if you still need a ride I'll be glad to take you home."

"John, chivalry never dies as long as there are men like you still out there."

Lynn was sucking up real good. All night while Lynn was romancing John, John was looking at Jill and Jill at John. Jill came over and said, "John, I'm ready for that dance." John and Jill felt instant sparks flying.

"Jill, would you like to have dinner with me one evening soon? I have a very important business meeting at 8:00 in the morning, and unfortunately, I won't be able to stay late."

"If you disappear after the cake is cut, I'll understand," Jill said.

The dance ended and John kissed Jill on the cheek, and went back to sit at the bar. As John finished his drink, he started feeling dizzy. John said, "I need some air. I don't feel so good." John got up and Lynn was there to grab his arm.

"Let me help you, she said." He rested his arm on her shoulder and Lynn held tightly to his waist. Just then Jill turned around and saw them leave together. Jill was very disappointed and said to her girlfriend, "Men! They're all the same. Oh well, you can forget that one. Let's enjoy my party."

Outside Lynn said, "Let me drive your car. You're not well." John got in the car and Lynn drove him home. She helped him in and put him on the couch. Five minutes later he passed out and couldn't remember a thing when he got up the next morning.

When he awoke, he was groggy and the front door was wide open. His Rolex and money were gone. He immediately called the police.

The police told him to get out of the house until they got there. They were concerned that someone might still be in the house.

John went outside to find that his car was missing. The police determined that Lynn had put a drug in his drink while he was dancing with Jill. She then brought him home and robbed him.

A couple of days later John called Jill and told her what happened. She was in shock and didn't know who the blonde was. In fact, no one knew who she was. Her story was a lie.

The police told John that there were reports of a pretty blonde who was crashing parties, drugging her targets and then robbing them.

Lucille Fordin

John and Jill dated every day for the next year. What a great couple they made. They flew to Las Vegas and got married. After what happened at Jill's birthday party, you can't blame them for wanting to celebrate their glorious occasion alone.

Chapter Sixteen:
Who Do You Trust?

One Saturday morning in September, Gigi, my Latin hairdresser, refused to do a client named Lori. Lori had a cold. Gigi called me over to her station. As I approached the two of them, I could hear them arguing, and Lori was refusing to get out of the chair. Gigi was hysterical and I had to calm her down fast. She was booked solid.

I said to Gigi, "Calm down. The whole salon is listening to you. I'll do Lori's hair, if it's okay with Lori."

Lori was really mad. "Lucy, I'm a steady customer for four years," she said loudly. I let Gigi do my hair when she had a cold, and now she doesn't want to do my hair. It's not fair. I don't want this bitch to ever again touch me. It's not my fault she had a fight with her boyfriend last night. She told me she hates all men. She's taking her anger out on me, and I have a date tonight. Lucy, please do my hair."

I told Lori to go to my station and that I'd be there in a moment. I had to talk to Gigi. I told Gigi she could have put a paper mask on Lori or herself. Taking her personal problems out on a client is not acceptable in my salon. Gigi threatened to quit, saying, "No one tells me what to do, you or my boyfriend."

I told Gigi, "You need to take a coffee break and calm down. I know you don't mean what you're saying."

As I walked away, I could feel my stomach turning sour. Could she be mad enough to quit her job over a man? I felt very insecure at that moment, and went to do Lori's hair.

I finished Lori and as I walked by Jessie's manicure station, I could hear Gigi telling her what happened the night before. She said her

Lucille Fordin

boyfriend had a cold and she didn't want to get sick, so she told him to leave. He slammed the door on her and left.

Jessie said, "I hate men. I didn't get laid last night either. My boyfriend wasn't in the mood."

Mila said, "I love men."

Everyone was verbally attacking Mila for loving men and called her a jerk. The salon was in a hate mood and I knew I had to do something to change it.

I said, "Girls, you know you don't hate men. We can't live without them, but you do need a lot of strength to be in a relationship."

A conversation about men, sex, and age started with myself, the employees and the clients.

Michele was having a manicure with Jessie and other clients were listening when she said, "I've been married five times and only one of the five was good in bed. I ended up marrying him twice. Louis was number two and four. I guess that's why he cheated; he could never get enough sex. I live now on those memories. Louis died of a heart attack and my new husband is eighty-two and can't get a hard on. I'm only seventy-eight and I need sex. I'm not dead yet."

Jessie laughed and told Michele she only looked seventy and should get a boyfriend.

Rhonda was getting a manicure with Mila and said abruptly, "All men are pigs. At least your memories are good ones. My ex was screwing my best friend. I prayed every night for him to become impotent. That's the best punishment a man could ever get."

I said to Rhonda, "Don't stop now. You got our attention. Did his stupid penis stay hard or soft?"

"Lucy, my ex, Lou, stayed soft with me, but kept getting hard with my best friend. Once a pig, always a pig."

Wilma was sitting next to Rhonda and waiting for a manicure when she jumped in and said, "You're both right. I've been married thirty years and I don't like sex, but my husband is wonderful. I was raped by my cousin when I was twelve."

"I can top that, Wilma," Janet said. "My parents put me in a foster home when I was thirteen because I told my dear mother her brother was raping me. Then my father raped me, and no one would believe me. I got into a lot of trouble after that."

Lori jumped in and said, "You women don't know what tragedy is. My daughter was killed in a car accident. My husband left me shortly after that for a man."

Linda said, "You haven't lived until you've ended up in a hotel room with a man who proceeds to take his hair off, and then his teeth out. He tried gumming me to death. Needless to say I threw up all over him."

We looked at each other and got hysterical laughing. "Now Lucy, it's your turn. Tell us some disgusting story that happened to you."

"Girls, I've heard enough. You don't need to hear my stories. We all had things happen to us. Ladies, a woman told me one day by the time we figure out who has the strength to get on top, it's soft again."

"Darla, we could all use a good story every now and then, especially now that we're all depressed."

"Okay," Darla said. "I met Adam when I was twenty. I was a virgin. So who knew the difference between good or bad? I fell deeply in love with Adam. We experimented together and the sex was great. When we were in our thirties, our lives were so busy starting a new business and raising our children, nothing felt the same. Sex became boring and infrequent. When we were in our fifties the kids were on their own and we traveled a lot. That's when the sex got better. It was like we met each other for the first time. Now we're in our sixties and all I can tell you is that it's slower and better."

Gigi turned to me, apologized, and said, "I feel better now, Lucy. My life's not so bad." We hugged and she went back to work.

The women opened the book on their lives and told me the rest of their stories in private, over a period of time.

Michele had been coming to the salon for eighteen years. Her first husband was a self-made millionaire. Michele had four children with him. He died at forty from a brain tumor. Michele was rich and alone, a dangerous combination. Her second husband Louis was very handsome and a playboy. Louis had very little money. Michele didn't care because they stayed in bed having sex most of the time, while her nanny took care of the children.

Lucille Fordin

One day Louis said, "I have business to take care of and I have to stay in Boston for two days." So Michele decided to go to New York City to do some shopping. Call it bad luck or call it fate, but while she was deciding where to have lunch she sees Louis and a young girl in her twenties getting out of a cab and walking into a restaurant holding hands.

"Business," she said to herself. "I'll kill that little bitch Louis is with, then I'll kill him." It took her about thirty minutes to come back to reality when she decided to approach them. As she entered the restaurant she could see Louis and his date sipping champagne and kissing. She went crazy and walked over to the table. "Business, Louis?" she said. "Oh you must have meant monkey business. By the way, who's the bimbo you're with?"

The girl at the table asked, "Louis, do you know this woman?" Louis never said a word.

"Louis? Tell your bimbo who I am, you creep. You're spending my money on this little bitch? I'm his wife; who the hell are you?"

"His wife? But Louis isn't married. Why don't you leave before you make a complete fool of yourself?"

"Here's a newsflash, Louis. I'm filing for a divorce. I'll send you your clothes. Don't ever set foot in my house again." Michele picked up the champagne and started pouring it all over the girl's head. "Now, how do you like your pretty little bitch?" she said. Michele walked away with a smile on her face and immediately shut off all Louis's credit cards with a few well-placed calls.

Michele moved to Florida after the divorce was final and met her third husband at a party. Johnny was a great guy, but thirty years older. He died five years later and left Michele everything. Now Michele was a multi-millionaire.

Louis had the audacity to show up at the guy's funeral, but over the next year, Louis proved he was a changed man and they got married again. Michele was happier than I ever saw her. Money didn't matter. Louis had a free hand on everything. Sex was good and Louis was known as quite the gorgeous stud by everyone who knew them.

Going to Las Vegas became a regular diversion for Louis, and he was losing a lot of money. Louis apparently stayed faithful for two years but managed to lose at least one million dollars… that Michele knew about.

Their last trip to Las Vegas was the end of their marriage. Michele caught Louis cheating with a dancer and came home alone. Louis stayed in Las Vegas and married the showgirl.

Michele stayed alone for a long time. At age seventy she is married to her fifth husband—a very gentle, kind man who says yes to everything and anything Michele wants. She's happy once again.

Rhonda, on the other hand, got divorced at fifty-two and vowed never to get married again. Rhonda was very poor as a child and had four brothers and one sister. Rhonda and her sister had to learn to eat fast or her brothers would consume everything. To this day she eats like every meal is her last meal.

Rhonda went to school with a girl named Judy, who was her best friend for thirty-two years. Judy was sleeping with Rhonda's husband Lou for twenty years, and no one else ever knew until Judy's husband died. That's when Lou asked Rhonda for a divorce because he was in love with Judy.

Rhonda told me at the salon one day that when she got sick, Judy came over immediately.

"Judy had her sister take care of her family and she stayed with me for three days." But while Judy was making Rhonda soup, she was also screwing Lou.

"Lucy," Rhonda said, "when I think back to all the times I thought my best friend came running anytime I needed help, it was just an excuse for Judy and Lou to be alone together.

"One time we stayed at the beach with both our families. Lou and Judy would disappear for a couple of hours at a time. I didn't know then why every time we needed groceries or anything Lou would run the errand and Judy would always go to help. The pig was probably screwing her in our car, on the beach, and even in my own house. My best friend was my worst enemy and I never suspected a thing! I trusted her like a sister. When I told Judy, 'I think my husband is having an affair,' the whole time it was that bitch. For twenty years! Lucy, please don't ever trust your friends or anyone with your man. That's why I don't have any friends, or any men in my life. You can't trust anyone."

"Rhonda, my mother told me years ago to never leave your best friend alone with your husband. I used to argue with her and say, 'You

Lucille Fordin

don't trust anyone, but I can trust my friends.' Well, one day I found out she was right. My best friend went out on a date with one of my boyfriends. Do you know what she said when she got caught? 'I thought we were going to meet you, Lucy. He said you were in trouble.'

"Rhonda, you're right, I'll never trust anyone with my boyfriends again." I never forgot that pain. To this day I'm still cautious.

What kind of world has this become? If you can't trust your friends and you can't trust your family, then who do you trust?

Wilma was raped by her eighteen year-old cousin when she was twelve. For two years Wilma was raped until she got pregnant and had an abortion. Wilma's rapist cousin was her babysitter. She tried to tell her parents that she was old enough to stay home alone, but every time the adults went out together her cousin offered to visit and stay home with Wilma "so she would be safe." Wilma tried every excuse in the book without being direct about it. Her parents were of the old school and very square. She was convinced they'd never believe her. Two years later she got pregnant and had an abortion. The two families never spoke again. Wilma's family kept the secret and never prosecuted the cousin. She always blamed herself for destroying the family.

Saturday afternoon, the same day that Rhonda, Michele, Lori and Linda told me their stories, my client named Janet came in the salon for a haircut and blow and said to me, "I can't believe I can't get pregnant."

While I was doing her hair, I said, "Janet, I tried everything and couldn't get pregnant. I had artificial insemination twice and ended up with a chlamydia infection, so I quit."

"Lucy, did you ever think of adopting? There are a lot of kids who need homes."

"Janet, after listening to a lot of adults who say to me, 'I'm trying to find my real parents,' I just couldn't adopt. I could never live through the pain of a child I loved and raised saying to me, 'I have to find my real parents.'"

"Lucy, I'm going to tell you a story about myself. A lot of children end up in foster homes for different reasons. My uncle was raping me. When I told my mother about it, she called me a liar. My parents put me in a foster home to teach me a lesson. Great lesson I got! My foster father called me a whore and raped me, too. When I told my parents, they told me I'd never come home if I kept on lying, so they left me there.

I toughened up on the streets. I told my uncle if he ever decided to come near me again I'd kill him, and he knew I meant it.

"Lucy, I always prayed someone else would adopt me, someone like you who would care enough to give me the time and patience and love that I needed. Who knows how many children out there are in the same situation I was, or worse? They need good people to help them survive."

Janet made me think about adopting every time I saw her. I wanted children very badly, but at the time, my first marriage was falling apart. No time became the right time, and I ended up with a hysterectomy, a tragic day for me forever. I never did adopt.

Lori had double tragedy in a completely different direction. She was married for thirty years. Lori received a call one Saturday night that her only child was dead. She felt it should have been her son-in-law that got killed, not her daughter.

Lori came into the salon looking very depressed. I gave her my deepest sympathy and I told her I'd be ready for her in five minutes. She had her hair washed while I finished another client. Lori sat in my chair and immediately started talking and crying.

"Lucy, I just don't understand. Any time I go anywhere with my husband and we happen to have two cars, he's always sure to follow me home, but not my son-in-law. He always left Debbie behind."

"Lori, I'm puzzled. Why did they go to the party in separate cars?"

"Her husband Jay had to go to the office Saturday so he called Debbie and said, 'I'll have to meet you at the party. I'm running late.' Jay had no business working Saturday. He's a workaholic and he's never home. Jay was behind Debbie, following her. Then for some reason he passed her and took off like a bat out of hell. Debbie always drove cautiously. Jay would always say, 'Debbie, you drive like an old lady.' Everything with Jay had to be fast and furious.

"Jay was home in ten minutes, but Debbie never arrived. The police went to their house and told Jay there was a car accident. From what I understand a man ran a red light doing seventy miles an hour, killed my daughter and killed himself. I'm glad the drunk is dead but I blame my son-in-law for Debbie's death. He should have never left her alone that

Lucille Fordin

late at night. He should have been behind her, not in front of her. I'll never forgive him. Jay knew Debbie didn't like to drive at night, but Jay said he had to go back to the office on Sunday. He insisted Debbie drive the car home because he had no time to take her to retrieve it on Sunday.

I couldn't control my tears when I asked Lori, "How's your husband D.J. handling all of this?"

"Badly. He's very depressed and I don't know what to do. He's drinking a lot. He hasn't been coming home from work until after midnight. When I call, they tell me he left the office at seven. I've tried to talk to him, but he just won't talk about it. All I do is cry, all day and all night. Lucy, my beautiful daughter, is dead!" She was crying as she left the salon.

I was very depressed, but had to go back to work. It was awful every time a client complained about the coffee being too strong or having to wait ten minutes for a hairdresser. All I could think was, They don't know what real problems are if this is all that bothers them. I wanted to scream, but of course, I didn't. I'm a boss. I had to stay in control and I did until I closed the salon. I cried in the car all the way home. I couldn't get Lori out of my thoughts.

Six months went by and I hadn't seen Lori. I called and left messages once a month. I was very concerned about her. Two weeks after the last call I made, Lori came into the salon. "Hi, Lucy. Thanks for calling so much. I'm sorry I never returned your calls. I've had a lot of trouble with D.J. We're getting a divorce."

"A divorce? I don't understand. After a horrible tragedy? You need each other now, more than ever. Oh my God, Lori, I'm so sorry. If there's anything I can do to help you, please don't hesitate to call me."

"Lucy, don't be upset. D.J. is a cheating pig and I'm tired of being alone. Thirty years of marriage meant nothing to him. I never knew for sure; I guess I kept my eyes closed. All those nights he said he was working? He wasn't. He's a cheating pig. I'll never get married again."

"Lori, who's the woman that did this to you? It's usually someone they work with."

"You're right. It's an office affair, alright. It's DJ's secretary, Bob!"

"Bob? Oh my God, D.J. is gay? I can't believe it! Are you sure, Lori?"

"Oh, I'm sure. They're living together. D.J. came to me two months ago and told me he was leaving me because he was in love with someone else. Now that Debbie is gone, he couldn't keep his secret any longer. D.J. took his clothes and left."

"Lori, can I ask you a personal question?"

"Yes, Lucy."

"Did you ever have any idea that D.J. was gay? Couldn't you tell by his actions?"

"No, Lucy," Lori said as her face drooped with despair. "We would play games in the bedroom. I would put on his clothes and be the man, and then D.J. would put on my underwear and pretend he was the woman. We had great sex on our dress-up nights. I would have never believed he was gay. I still can't believe he's gay. I feel so stupid!"

"Lori, don't punish yourself. I hear plenty of stories in the salon about dress-up night for sex. You didn't have the problem; D.J. has the problem. He waited too long to come out of the closet. What a creep to do this to you now when you need him the most."

"I'm fine Lucy, honest. At least now I don't have to wonder what's wrong with me. I have always thought that it was me. The last ten years things haven't been good between us. Now I don't have to worry about him anymore. I'm getting help for myself and have no intentions of ever getting married again."

I couldn't believe what Lori told me that day. What a horrible time D.J. picked to come out of the closet. He saved himself and hurt Lori forever.

Linda's story was quite the opposite. She loved men and had no trouble picking up anyone she wanted. She was sixty and gorgeous, with blonde hair (thanks to me) and blue eyes.

Linda just finished getting a pedicure and needed time to dry her polish. I needed a coffee break, so I sat in the waiting area with Linda.

"Linda, aren't you glad I made you a blonde? You're beautiful. Your brown hair never got you so many dates."

"Yes, Lucy. Let me tell you about a date I had in California."

Linda loved to go on trips by herself. In Los Angeles she and met a guy named Fast Freddy. Freddy was about sixty-five and a big gambler.

Lucille Fordin

Linda was having a drink in the lounge of a fancy hotel when she met Freddy. He approached her and said, "Hi, my name is Freddy. Are you here alone? Can I buy you a drink?"

"Yes, you may. I saved this seat for a handsome guy like you. My name is Linda."

The two of them talked and danced for hours. It seemed like Freddy was well known and liked by all. The bartender was calling him Fast Freddy. Linda said, "Why is he calling you Fast Freddy? You must pick up a lot of women in this lounge."

"No, I don't Linda. I'm not sure if you would believe me, so I want you to ask the bartender what that name means."

The next time the bartender brought a drink, he said, "Can I get you anything else, Fast Freddy?"

"It's okay, Joe. You can tell the lady how I got my nickname."

"Well, miss, when Fast Freddy is at the crap table, the croupier can't keep up with him. He rolls the dice so fast he'd make your head spin. So that's why he's called Fast Freddy."

"Thanks, Joe, for telling me. I was sure it had something to do with women."

"I'm afraid not. Freddy usually sits alone. You must be a special lady."

"Thank you. My name is Fast Linda. Ha! Ha!" Joe walked away smiling.

"Linda, I'm leaving tomorrow. What can I do to convince you to spend this beautiful night with me? I have a bottle of Dom Perignon in my room. Would you like to share it with me?"

Linda was already pretty high and always adventurous. "Let's go, baby, I'm yours."

Linda used Fast Freddy's restroom first. She got undressed and slipped under the covers. Fast Freddy dimmed the lights and poured the champagne. They were both hotter than firecrackers . . . or is it pepper sprouts?

"I'll be back in a minute. I have to use the little boys' room," Freddy said. When he returned, his hair was gone.

"Freddy, I couldn't even tell that you were wearing a hairpiece."

"I hope you don't mind, Linda."

At this point Linda was so turned on that the hair, or lack of it, meant absolutely nothing to her.

"I'll show you how much I mind, Freddy. Come to me baby." They started making love and Freddy said. "I hope you don't mind, but I have one more thing to remove. Then I'll put you in heaven."

"Freddy, you're bone naked. What's left?"

Within a second Freddy took out his teeth and started gumming her to death. Freddy started chewing on her tongue.

"How gross!"

He chewed on her nipples and then looked up at her with spit dripping from his face and said, "Linda, isn't this the best sex you ever had? I can't bite you this way." Now whether it was the liquor or seeing him bald and feeling him with no teeth, Linda said, "I don't feel well." But Ol' Fast Freddy kept on a-goin'.

Freddy continued licking his way down her belly. Freddy almost made it to Linda's vulva when she threw up all over him.

I started laughing so hard that I was crying. Linda was choking from laughing. Clients who eavesdropped on Linda's story were laughing and grimacing. "Yuck!" they said.

I told Linda she was a better person than me. I would have thrown up the minute his teeth came out. I had to go back to work, and I felt as if I could never eat lunch again. Yuck!

The moral to Linda's story is: Keep you hair on your head and your teeth in your mouth if you want to keep your dinner down and your libido up.

Chapter Seventeen:
Like a Bunch of Dirty Old School Boys

It was October and time for daylight savings time to come to an end. I hate it when it gets dark early. It forces me to get some things done earlier instead of later.

When I arrived to open my salon that morning, I found a bouquet of dead flowers in front of the door with a note that said, "Get out of town, bimbo, or you'll end up like these flowers."

All I could think was that the shrimp had struck again. I picked up the phone and called Pepe at his salon. Pepe answered the phone, and I said, "Pepe, I've had enough of your shit, dead flowers and threats. You're not the Mafia. You're a jealous punk. Back off or you'll be sorry."

He didn't deny anything and started screaming at me. "That's nothing. I know a lot of people, you bitch. I'm going to make a phone call right now to a powerful man to blow up your salon."

I very quickly replied in a tough, street-smart voice, "Now you did it, loser. Would you like to see who can get the job done first?" I slammed the phone down in his ear. I'm glad I taped the whole conversation. I was very nervous and I must admit, scared. I couldn't help but wonder if Pepe was crazy enough to pay someone to blow up my salon. I decided to call Gino, a client of mine. I explained the situation and played the tape for him. I didn't know for sure, but I heard rumors that Gino was connected to the mob.

Gino said, "Don't worry about anything, Lucy. You take good care of me and my family at the salon, and I'll take care of business for you. Everything will be okay."

Two hours later, Gino called me at the salon. "Lucy, don't worry about nothing. It's all taken care of. Pepe called a friend of mine to try to

Lucille Fordin

do what he said he would do, but I put a stop to it. Because he's such a nice guy, I sent him a special present. He should be getting it just about now. He will never be able to do that thing... you know what I mean?"

"Yes." I couldn't thank Gino enough and told him the next day in the salon that haircuts for him and his family were on the house.

He thanked me and said, "That's not necessary. I hate that punk. He's got a big mouth. He borrows money and tells people he's part of our family. He's a wannabe wiseguy."

I took care of Gino's family in the salon during their next visit. The next day, Gino had lunch delivered for me and my employees with a thank you note for my kindness to his family.

Gino's business with the mob was a bad thing, but I think he's one of the nicest, most generous guys I know.

The next day I received a phone call from Pepe. He was nervous and was talking very fast. "Lucy, I'm sorry for bothering you. I wasn't serious. It was only a joke. I have a hot temper. I'm so sorry. I will never bother you again, sweetheart."

"Okay." I accepted his apology. When I hung up I had a feeling he wasn't done yet with his games. I knew he couldn't put a contract out on me or the salon, but I could tell that the shrimp thought that he could outsmart anyone. He had a cocky attitude, but this time he had outsmarted himself.

That evening I was cleaning the waiting area at the salon for the twenty-fifth time that day. I had bad memories of the twelve years I couldn't afford a maid in the salon. I help the maid clean when it's busy, doing my clients, greeting people, handling little arguments between clients and other clients waiting too long, and clients arguing with the hairdressers. I needed to be super woman some days. The cause of these arguments was being late and two famous words, I'm next. Certain clients arrived five to fifteen minutes late for their appointments, which made everyone run late by the end of the day. Three gentlemen were sitting in the waiting room discussing where they were going for dinner if their wives ever got out of the salon. It was 7pm; the salon was quiet and nearly empty.

My waiting area seats ten. I have a round table with chairs around the table for eating, drinking coffee, or reading magazines. The main topic of conversation in Miami was, "Which restaurant are we going to?", or who has the best doctor.

Marlene's been coming to me for three years. Her husband Morris is a loudmouth know-it-all, happily married for fifty-five years.

Betty's been going to Renaldo for five years. Her husband Jason is a sweet, gentle man. They've been married for fifty-two years.

Evelyn's been going to Gigi for seven years.

Jacob seems like a decent guy, but I notice him looking at the other women a lot.

The men were talking loudly when I heard this three-way conversation.

Morris said, "Renaldo has a great job working with all these women. You're single, Brent. Wouldn't you like to bang that Gigi?"

"She's one hot mama."

"Jason, are you sure you never cheated on Betty?"

"Morris, go take a cold shower. You're an old man."

"I'm not old, I just look old. Look at the way Gigi moves around the chair, Brent. What a cute ass she has."

I stopped doing Marlene's hair, and said, "Guys, guys! I can hear you. You're going to get yourselves in trouble."

Morris said, "We know, but it's fun. Hurry up, Lucy, and get my wife's hair done."

As I turned away, Jason said, "That Lucy's a real woman."

"Jason, you're no better than me", Morris blurted out.

"Morris, I can look, can't I? Betty would cut off my balls if I ever cheated . . . and got caught."

"Look what happened to Brent. His girlfriend caught him cheating, and being the nice lady she is, Evelyn never said a word! One day, as Brent left his apartment, there was a sign on his front door, 'This is the home of a cheater.' I'm sure it had to be Evelyn who put the sign up."

Brent said, "Jason, I don't think Evelyn did it. Would she still be with me if she knew I cheated? Besides, we're not married. I can do whatever I want."

Jason, the quiet one said, "Brent you're a lucky man. Betty would have cut my balls off and stuffed them down my throat!"

Lucille Fordin

The three of them were laughing like a bunch of dirty old school boys when Morris said, "Marlene has Lucy do her hair. She's a nice girl and she works hard. I bet she gives a good bang. She doesn't look smart enough to run her own business, though."

"Jason, how smart do you have to be to play with hair all day? I'm single; I could help her run the business. I'm getting tired of Evelyn anyway and Lucy is a good catch. Is she married? Find out for me, Morris."

"Okay, I'll ask Marlene."

"Brent, you don't have a pot to piss in. Don't you think you should hang on to Evelyn? She pays for everything."

"Don't start, Morris. I'm worth it. Where could she find another stud like me?"

"Ah, the Viagra king has spoken. Jason, you wish Betty was as hot as Evelyn."

"My Betty is a good woman and a good cook. Marlene has flowers growing out of her oven. When was the last time she cooked for you or gave you a blow job?"

Just then Jason said, "That reminds me of a joke I heard at the golf course: Go-um in teepee take-um off panties. Don't have time to chew fat, just have time to cum and go."

"Jason, that's a good one. I don't have time to cum; I'm busy going all night. Those days are over. The bathroom is the hot spot in our apartment now. Besides, Brent is getting enough action for all of us."

"Here come the women. Let's see where and what our darlings want to eat. Maybe if we're lucky, boys, they'll say, 'We want to eat you!'"

I said goodnight to all of them and locked the door fast before the Three Stooges decided to come back. I was very glad another day was over.

Chapter Eighteen:
My Sweet Karate Blocks

Didn't I say I'd never get married again? Didn't I say I hated all men? Well guess what? I started dating again.

A lovely lady named Maggie came into the salon one day and said, "Lucy I want you to take my Country Club card so you can meet someone great. You have to be a member or guest to get in. You said you couldn't afford to join the club, but how do you expect to meet someone decent who can take care of you financially?"

"Thanks, but no thanks. Thanks for thinking of me."

"Lucy, you have to make your own luck. I'm on my third husband and I've had money all my life. Believe me, I'd rather be depressed with money than without money. You've always been so nice to me, and I want to do something nice for you. Please use it, and when it expires in eight months you can get your own card if you want. You'll love it. My husband has his card for us to use."

I realized Maggie was right. I got so excited I kissed her and said thanks. This really changed my life, and I'll never forget what Maggie did for me. I also found out after living in Florida that Jewish people didn't have all the money in the world, like most people think. I know plenty of rich Catholics and Protestants from all over the world who come into my salon. I was scared I'd sound stupid or not fit in because my knowledge couldn't compare to what most of these intelligent people knew. I had common sense and a lot of street knowledge, but I lacked book knowledge. The main thing is that I treated everyone the way I wanted to be treated, and that is with respect.

Working in Miami and being around wealthy people had changed my thinking. I wasn't scared of rich people anymore. They were trying to sur-

Lucille Fordin

vive just like me, but on a different level. Believe me, their lives could be a lot tougher than most. Everyone was always trying to take something from them. That's a difficult way to live, with everyone wanting something from you.

I worked all day and made arrangements with a couple of friends of mine, who were all club members, to go to the Country Club that night. I was nervous, but I got dressed and met my friends. It was hard to date after fifteen years of marriage; I lost my nerve.

Anita was testing me. "This is like taking a virgin into a den of wolves." That made me real calm! My palms were sweating, and I never sweat. We arrived at the club, went to the bar, and the bartender asked, "What can I get you three lovely ladies?

The club was beautiful. I had never been in a high-class club before. The band was playing a love song. People were dancing and talking. There were plush chairs and couches for people to sit on in the cocktail lounge. The bar sat around fifty people.

Anita said to the bartender, "I'll have you, cutie, with two olives." My mouth dropped open and my eyes opened up wide. We all burst out laughing. We were the only ones laughing and having a good time. Soon all the men started shifting our way. A gorgeous man with thick white hair sent a drink to me. I accepted, then smiled and said thanks. The more we laughed, the more everyone sent drinks over. Then they asked if they could join us. Soon we knew everyone and I felt at home.

I ended up dating that gorgeous man for six months. Marty was Jewish and fifty-eight years old. He was retired. A perfect gentleman. He wined and dined me out in the open. I broke up with him when I found out from a client that he was married. Marty didn't deny his marriage when I confronted him, but this was not what I wanted. I could never trust him again. I don't know what I was thinking at the time, but I learned a lesson. I refuse to date married men. I thought I'd be safe from the creeps of the world because I was in a Country Club. None of these people were poor, so I thought their morals would be sterling. I found out that some worked hard to get where they were, but that others inherited their money and were mostly lazy, depressed, and spoiled rotten.

The club was my new hangout. I was sitting at the Club bar one night and looked over at a beautiful blonde woman with diamonds on her fingers as big as golf balls. She looked around sixty years old and was with a handsome guy who looked forty. They were kissing, and all I could think is, "Good for her." I personally never liked dating younger guys. I've always believed that men were real men when they were older.

As I was thinking what a lovely couple they were, I noticed her squirming around in her chair. When I looked again, I saw that he had his hand up her dress and was playing with her. Everyone started to giggle and look. It never stopped them. She thought she was hot stuff. She was nothing more than a tramp. I felt embarrassed just to be there. I felt like a piece of trash just being in their presence. I paid my bill and left feeling very insecure. I hated dating. It scared me not knowing who anyone was, or if they were telling me the truth about themselves.

One evening I was having dinner with a date at the Villa Riviera, an excellent Italian restaurant, when two limousines pulled up. A man got out of the first limo and ten guys got out of the second and followed him into the restaurant. Two guys sat at the table, four guys sat in front of them, and four guys sat behind them. It was obvious they were the first man's bodyguards. They kept looking around the restaurant and never took their eyes off the man they came in with. But who were these people? All of them were whispering, and no one was ordering food, but food was automatically put on their tables. Four waiters were immediately at their sides. One of the gentlemen looked up at me and smiled. Well, naturally, I smiled and turned away. I could feel him staring at me. The next day I saw Mr. Smiles on TV. He was apparently the son of a major Mafia family don. I love strong, good-looking men. I've always been attracted to them, and them to me. Now if I had not been with a date, look where I might have ended up. Not again, thank God.

A week later I was invited to a party—my first real party with rich and influential people. I went out and bought a new outfit. I was so nervous. I knew nothing about politics, stocks, investments, etc. When someone would ask what kind of business I owned, I'd say a hair salon. They would say, "It figures. What a joke! That's not a business. All you do is play with hair all day." Some would laugh in my face. At times like that, I wished I were a man. I'd like to see one of them come and work one day in the salon and see if all we do is play with hair. For some stupid reason, men get all the respect.

Lucille Fordin

As I pulled into the driveway of the three million dollar house on the water, I saw three valets waiting to park the cars. I could hear my knees knocking. A man opened the door and said, "Good evening, madame. May I see your invitation, please?"

The house was magnificent. I could see food, drinks, and servants everywhere. There was elegance galore. I asked Grace, my client who was giving the party, if I could walk around and look at the rest of the house.

She said, "Sure, but the bedrooms and the office are locked up because after the last party I gave, I was missing a lot of little things."

"No way. Only poor people steal," I replied.

"You've got a lot to learn, Lucy. People are people, rich or poor."

I went up a winding staircase, which led to a giant bar with at least fifty elegant people sitting around it. In the next room there was great disco music playing. People were dancing all over the place. I went down the hall and opened the door and guess what I found? People sitting around a table snorting cocaine. Someone said to me, "It's on the house, compliments of the host." I was shocked and said, "Thanks, I already had mine," and shut the door fast. I wanted nothing to do with cocaine.

I spent my whole life getting out of the slums, where drugs were everywhere. Being here was no different than being back there. The only difference was the furniture, which was a lot nicer, and they had servants. I was very disappointed to say the least. I wanted to leave.

Upstairs drugs, downstairs violins playing. A man asked me to slow dance and I accepted.

"What's your name?"

"Lucy. What's yours?"

"Gregory." He pulled me in close to his body. "Are you here alone?"

"Yes. I own the hair salon that Grace goes to." Gregory's hands were getting real friendly real fast. I was doing my sweet karate blocks to stop him when he said, "I'm here with my wife, but I always dance with the girls. My wife is cool with my toys. Would you like to be one of my toys?"

Just then a girl at the top of the stairs near the bar took off her blouse and threw her bra over the railing. Everyone was looking up. Some people laughed, some smiled, some just shook their heads. One second later it was as if nothing had ever happened. Everyone went back to what they were doing.

Gregory pulled me close again and put one hand on my breast. Well, that was enough for me. I pulled away and as soon as I found Grace, I told her what happened.

Grace said, "Lucy! Girls would die just to have Gregory make them an offer. You should feel special. Try to enjoy the party." As Grace walked away, I thought, "Special! She thinks that was special? I'm in trouble now. I have to get out of here. This is not for me." When no one was looking I ran out the front door and went home.

I sat down, had a cigarette, and thought about what the hell had just happened. My excitement and high from having been invited to the party were ruined. I was so depressed it felt as if I were hitting bottom again. Grace was a sweet, nice woman when she came in the salon. At the party she was as loose as a goose, a real playgirl. I wasn't going to anymore of Grace's parties.

If any of you think the lifestyle of the rich and famous is the answer to life, you're wrong. There's just as much twisted crap going on in their lives as there is in ours. It's no different, really. So try not to be bitter because you're not rich. Instead, thank God for what you have.

Chapter Nineteen:
He Loves Me Like My Mother Loved Me

The salon was very busy, and when I looked up a very handsome guy was standing at the front desk. All I could think was, "Wow!" He was on his way to get a manicure and I heard him say to me, "Hi Lucy, it's Jonathan. Jonathan Bain, Joanne Bain's son from New York." Joanne Bain and her family had been my clients for fifteen years.

"I'm sorry, I didn't recognize you. You lost some weight and your tan is very nice. You look terrific. It's been about five years since I last saw you. What are you doing in Florida?"

"Visiting my mother. Lucy, I'm fifty-five now. How old are you?"

"I'm thirty-nine, almost forty."

"Did you ever have the kids you wanted, Lucy?"

"No, but I sure did try. I'm also divorced now. My brother Joe got married and my sister Roxanne married a great guy. She has two darling sons. My nephews are my life, just like your three children are your life. It's nice to see you again, Jonathan. Enjoy your manicure." As he walked away, all I could think was, "Wow!"

That night I went to the Country Club with my friends and Jonathan walked in with a date. He sat down at the bar next to me. He said, "Hi, Lucy," then introduced me to his date. We were all talking back and forth, having a good time. Always the hairdresser, I couldn't help but think what a beautiful head of hair that man had. His piercing blue eyes sparkled in the lights. I had no intention of intruding on him with his date. I believe you should never flirt with anyone's date or husband. I know I wouldn't like it if someone flirted with mine

Lucille Fordin

Jonathan was dancing all night. He was a perfect gentleman. He gave his date the respect she deserved. But every once in a while we would both glance over at each other and smile.

Later in the evening, someone accidentally bumped me and my purse fell on the floor. Jonathan bent over to pick it up at the same time I did and his hand touched mine. We stopped and looked into each other's eyes and guess what happened? I felt those damn tingles again. My mouth dropped open and nothing would come out. We both said, "I got it." All I could think was, "Wow!"

Jonathan called the bartender over and paid for everything. He said, "Goodnight, ladies, you're on your own. Be careful driving home." We stayed for a little while and then left.

I was driving my friend Rhoda home, who is also a client, and she never stopped talking about how good-looking Jonathan was and what she would have done if she were me, "to take him away from his date." In the beginning, his date was congenial. By the end of the evening, the blonde bombshell was intimidated, and the more she drank, the ruder she became.

The next day Jonathan's mother, Joanne Bain, came in to get her hair done and said, "Hi, Lucy. Jonathan said he saw you last night at the club. Do you go there often?"

"Joanne, I never go in the middle of the week. I usually go on Sunday night, but for some reason I just had to go out last night."

Sunday night Jonathan showed up at the Country Club alone.

I was sitting at the bar with my three friends, when he came up to us.

"Hi, Lucy. Would you mind if I joined you?"

I was glad Jonathan showed up. I was excited and nervous when I said, "Girls, do we mind if a gorgeous guy joins us?" Before I could finish the sentence, they were pulling a bar stool out for him.

Jonathan bought us all a drink. He spoke about the beach, stocks, his children, and told us a few jokes. I was so amazed at how intelligent, kind, and cute he was. At one point his leg accidentally touched mine, and I felt those damn tingles again. I instinctively moved over. He must have thought he did something wrong because of how quickly I moved away, but I didn't know what was happening to me.

Jonathan just smiled at me and said, "Lucy, would you like to have lunch with me tomorrow? Can I call you in the morning to make arrangements?"

"Absolutely." The next day when we got back from lunch I invited him into my place for coffee. It was as if we had known each other all our lives. At the door Jonathan said, "Would it be all right if I kissed you?"

As his lips touched mine, I felt my whole body tingling. He was so soft and gentle. We both pulled back, looked into each other's eyes, and fell back into kissing each other like there was no tomorrow. Jonathan finally pulled away and said, "Wow, was it the same for you?"

"Wow, and yes, you may call me anytime."

"Would tonight for dinner be too soon?"

That was the start of the most perfect and trusting relationship I ever had with a man. Jonathan never looked at another woman when he was with me. He was kind, considerate, and wanted to help me anyway he could. He always opened doors for me, and we would talk for hours. He never made me feel stupid. He made me feel proud of my accomplishments. Eight months later Jonathan moved to Florida and we were married. I was happier than I had ever been. This is going to be hard to explain, but he loved me like my mother loved me. There's no other way to put it, and nothing else to say about it. It was a shame that she never got to meet him.

My adopted stepmother Sandy was a magistrate. I wanted her to perform the services. She did a beautiful job. It brought tears to all of us. There wasn't a dry eye in the room. We had the ceremony in my home, with only his family, my family and a few close friends present. Fifty people altogether. We spent a lot of time driving back and forth to the airport in three days, until the last family member went home. Jonathan was the second best thing besides Sandy to come into my life. I love him to death to this day.

Chapter Twenty:
You're Italian, You Must Know Someone

It was October 31st. My Halloween party was only one day in the salon, a time to go crazy and be anyone you wished. I had decorated the entire salon with pumpkins, witches, and black cats. The employees come to work in elaborate costumes. I always tried to be something funny, so that year I was a cow. My udders were poking everyone all day as I hugged them. We never stopped laughing. Each employee makes a special dish from their country of origin. Our international buffet was a big hit. All of our clients throughout the week were invited to the party, and they all showed up for some fun or was it the free buffet? I chose to believe it was for the fun.

Mrs. Samuels was eating the lasagna I made, and said, "Lucy, I need help. I want to be a blonde."

Mrs. Samuels was a beautiful, sixty-five-year-old brunette. She got my attention, and I said, "Okay, so you want to go bald for Halloween."

She showed no reaction to my statement and said, "I just found out that my husband is having an affair with his secretary, who is thirty-five and blonde. I can't let my husband know that I know, but that bitch isn't getting him from me. He's a sixty-eight-year-old fool. Maybe I should have him killed. You're Italian, you must know someone." Then she started to cry. "Why would he do this to me? I'm so depressed."

I ran to the front desk to get a Kleenex for Mrs. Samuels and had the maid bring her a cup of coffee while I mixed the bleach for her hair. I prayed her hair didn't break. Everyone's hair reacts to bleach a little differently. Some hair is stronger than others. Mrs. Samuels had normal hair, not fine or thin, but to play it safe, I put conditioner in the bleach and used a conditioner after the color.

Lucille Fordin

I sat Mrs. Samuels in the hair dye area while her hair was processing. I had another client in my chair and could see Mrs. Samuels sobbing the whole time. I finished blowing my client's hair and went to check Mrs. Samuels' hair. All I could think was, please don't let her hair break. She'll kill me if she ends up bald. Her color was finished, and much to my surprise, no breakage had occurred at all. I made her a platinum blonde.

While I was blowing her hair, I suggested she try to make him fall in love with her all over again. After forty years, things can get pretty routine in a relationship. I had the makeup artist do her makeup, and then she was a beautiful platinum blonde.

I said, "Mrs. Samuels, you're lovely. Just look in the mirror and remember who you are inside. Oh, and go buy a negligee. Make his favorite meal and make love to him as if you were a teenager."

She laughed and said, "Okay Lucy, but if that doesn't work, will you please find me someone who will kill him?"

She reverted back into a depressed state, and said, "I'm rich. I'll pay anything. Please help me. You know everybody."

Just to calm her down, I said, "I'll ask around. Now go home and screw him to death. You're beautiful."

"You're right, I'm beautiful and no one is taking my husband. I'll see you next week."

The following week Mrs. Samuels told me that she went home and cooked him his favorite meal. She gave her servants the night off. At eight o'clock her husband came in the door and just stood there with his mouth open, looking at her in her black negligee and blonde hair. With his eyes bulging out, he said, "What's all this? Did I miss our anniversary or are you just flipping your lid? What did you do to your hair? Are you crazy?"

She walked over to him and kissed him and said, "I did this all for you because I love you. Can't you just enjoy it? After forty years I thought a change would be good."

They sat down to a candle lit dinner. It was just like when they were starting out together except they were eating filet mignon instead of ground meat. After dinner she said, "Come with me. I have a hot bath ready for you and then I have a surprise."

The ungrateful Mr. Samuels said, "It's late and I'm tired. I don't want any more surprises. I have to be at the office early tomorrow."

She didn't give up, "You soak in the tub, honey, and relax. I know you're tired; you were two hours late coming home tonight. I'm sure you were really busy."

Finally, after an hour, Mr. Samuels came out of the bath, and she had candles lit everywhere. She was ready to attack when he said, "I told you I was tired," and sat down on the bed. She still didn't give up. She reached over to kiss him goodnight and he didn't pull away. So she made love to him like never before. She said it was glorious.

The next morning he woke up and said, "Make an appointment with the psychologist. I do believe you're losing your ever-loving mind. You're acting like a whore. And another thing: Change your hair back. You must have a boyfriend because you look like a tramp." He stormed out the door saying, "Don't expect me for dinner. I have a business appointment."

She called me immediately to get her hair redone.

"Hello Lucy, I want my hair colored back to brown," she sobbed. "I need to talk to you. I'm coming in today."

I tried to tell her another dye job so soon could break all of her hair off, but she just wouldn't listen to me.

Mrs. Samuels came to the salon an hour later and said, "I'm so sorry. At least you tried. You can't be blamed. You gave it your best shot.

"I want him killed, Lucy, and that blonde bitch too. Did you find me someone who can do the job?"

I had to think fast. "The man is out of town for a month." I figured by then she would cool off and change her mind.

"I don't want his kids to know that their father is a pig," she said.

I suggested she call her therapist. Mrs. Samuels went to her therapist every day for the next week. She had her hair done every week, and she seemed to be doing well. She came in for her regular weekly appointment but she was wild with anger. I never saw this sweet woman so enraged. She had found bills for jewelry and also discovered he was paying for a condo for his girlfriend.

I had wrongly assumed she had forgotten about the hit man.

"You have to help me, Lucy. I want him killed."

Lucille Fordin

I tried to convince her to leave him instead of doing something stupid that would land her in jail and ruin her life and her kids' lives, but she kept insisting.

"Mrs. Samuels, please calm down. I'm not going to let you do something that stupid. Forget about the hit man."

"Lucy, I love you. I don't want you to get in any trouble because of me. I'm going to the doctor's right now." She made a hair appointment for next week and appeared to be calm as she left.

Needless to say, Mrs. Samuels didn't go to the doctor's. She went home and got her gun, which she kept for protection. She then had her chauffeur drive her to the mistress's condo. Her husband's car was there. She entered with some keys she found lying around her house. The girlfriend opened the door for her. She found her husband in her bed. She went crazy shooting at them. She shot her husband in the arm. The girlfriend made it into the bathroom and locked the door. Bullets were flying everywhere.

Mrs. Samuels finally dropped to the floor and started crying. She was in a mental hospital for a year. Her husband didn't prosecute. Should we give this guy a medal for only destroying her and not putting her in jail? I don't think so.

I went to the hospital the following week to do her hair, but all she wanted was her husband. She acted as if the affair and the shooting spree had never happened.

Mr. Samuels eventually got rid of the girlfriend and took care of his wife. What a price to pay for being in love.

Slowly I found out that rich people's problems were no different than poor people's problems. The only difference, obviously, was that they lived in bigger houses and had more money. I always believed having money made you happier. Well ding dong, I was wrong again.

One week after Mrs. Samuel's recovery, a beautiful Colombian girl came into the salon. She was a model — a tall, thin, beautiful, classy, sweet, good-hearted redhead with the longest legs I've ever seen in my life. Maria was twenty-five and became a good client of the salon for three years.

She said, "Lucy, you have to hide me. Someone's following me."

Maria was shaking all over. I quickly hid Maria in my office. Ten minutes later I said, "Maria, I don't see anyone who looks suspicious, nor did anyone come in asking for you. What's going on?"

"My husband caught me kissing my photographer. He said he was going to kill me."

"Maria, should I call the police?"

"No! No! No! If you do, he'll really kill me. You don't know my husband. He's crazy with jealousy. Lucy, I don't know how this happened. I love my husband. If it weren't for him, I wouldn't even be a model. He saved my life, but you should have seen this gorgeous Italian Adonis."

"We were in the middle of a photo shoot. He was snapping my picture and the music was really sensual and loud. I was so into the moment when he came close to me and I looked into his eyes and he looked into mine that we leaned into each other and kissed. It was completely spontaneous, Lucy. Then Roberto walked in.

"I told him it was just a kiss for the pictures."

Roberto screamed at us. "'I'll kill you and your boyfriend!' he said.

"I ran out the door and drove here. You were only two blocks away. I was sure he was following me, but I guess I lost him. He needs time to calm down. Then I'll try to explain things to him."

Maria was still shaking. Of course she was also half naked in her slinky black negligee. I gave her a dye gown to put on over her negligee. Maria had a beautiful body. I couldn't stop looking at her, and so did everyone else as she ran through the salon. It was like a show. All you could hear were remarks like, "Wow!", "Holy Mackerel!", and "Who's that?"

I said, "Maria, look at the good side of this. If Roberto had shown up twenty minutes later, you might have been in bigger trouble."

"No, I wouldn't have cheated on Roberto. Even though I thought about it for a second, I still wouldn't have done anything."

"Maria, maybe you have learned a lesson. You're young. You didn't do anything that anyone else wouldn't have done." Maria finally stopped crying and started to laugh.

"Now you have to convince Roberto that you're sorry and that you'll never do it again."

Lucille Fordin

A week went by and I heard from Maria that Roberto had beaten up the photographer. He also beat up Maria so that she couldn't work for a few months. I couldn't believe that they're back together again and in love. She actually felt she deserved the beating. She was convinced he'd never beat her again.

Why did Maria think that she deserved it? Roberto convinced her that she made him crazy. He loves her that much.

I've learned over the years that the beaters never stop. It only gets worse. So let's see if I have this right: Some men are crazy and some women are crazier.

Chapter Twenty-One:
Florida Grandmas Are Neither Baking Bread Nor Making Meatballs

It was Thanksgiving. I always think of my grandma this time of the year. For me, every Sunday was Thanksgiving at Grandma's, only there was no turkey, just lots of meatballs.

Every Sunday growing up in Pittsburgh, before we went to Grandma's house, we were allowed to play with our friends. When we'd arrive, Grandma would always be baking bread and cooking a giant pot of sauce and meatballs. We'd sneak into the kitchen and Joe, Roxanne and I would steal meatballs out of the pot. Grandma always knew what we were doing, but she pretended not to see us. We'd giggle and whisper and she'd always say week after week, "You better not be stealing my meatballs!" This was the type of grandmother I was used to.

Ever since Grandma died from cancer, anytime I was in trouble, I knew her spirit would help me. I could smell that foul odor that came from her body that was being eaten away from the cancer. Maybe it was my imagination, maybe not. A feeling of relief would come over me knowing my Grandma was with me in spirit.

Women in my salon, on occasion, told me that they had seen their dead husbands and children in a puff of smoke or at the bottom of their bed. Some saw shadows. Others heard noises. One woman found objects on the pillow next to her when she woke up in the morning. How could all of these occurrences be figments of our imaginations? Was it that we wanted our loved ones so badly that we caused these illusions ourselves?

Lucille Fordin

I guess we'll all find out the truth some day. I intend to ask my Grandma when I see her at the end of life on earth.

Florida grandmas are not baking bread nor making meatballs. Some have flowers growing out of their ovens. For many, breaking a fingernail is a major catastrophe. Most of them are model-thin and well-kept, with high heels and money to burn. Some have had up to five husbands. They're still out there, dancing and enjoying life up until the day they die. They have an attitude of independence. I don't wonder why. They don't have to worry where their next dollar is coming from. Plastic surgery is an every day occurrence. Implants, collagen injections, facelifts, lyposuction, tummy tucks and nose jobs help them to create the person they'd like to be. Most plastic surgeries turn out beautifully, but there's always that one lady who is not so fortunate. Grandma was sixty-seven when she died, and these women are older.

A sixty-eight year old woman came into the salon very excited that she was going to have a facelift. She saved her money for five years. She wasn't rich. She had the doctor pull her face as tight as he could. She had very thin skin and the swelling wouldn't go down.

One morning she woke up and found blood all over the bed. When she looked in the mirror, her face actually had split in two! The swelling made her face explode. They had to stitch her together and it was an unholy mess. She filed a lawsuit and had plenty of surgery and skin grafting. It took a couple of years to get her face back to normal again. She was awarded two million dollars.

What do you think she said when it was all over? "I'm rich now. It was well worth it."

Grandma was beautiful. Her wrinkles made her even more beautiful. She lived for her children and grandchildren. I loved spending time with her when she babysat me. Grandma always cooked whatever I wanted, and we would play games. When Grandma got tired, I would make her sit in a chair and pretend that I was a hairdresser. I was only four. I remember brushing her gray hair to make her feel better. I didn't know what cancer was at that time: I just knew I had to make her feel better. I always felt the need to please, to be her best little girl.

Marilyn Monroe was getting a manicure in Mila's chair. Did I say Marilyn Monroe? I meant Mrs. Betty Moss. Betty is seventy and a platinum blonde with gray roots. She had her lips tattooed red. They're swollen, and she's talking as if she has a bag of marbles in her mouth.

I said, "Betty, what happened to your lips?"

"Lucy, I had them tattooed so I don't have to put lipstick on anymore. They're a little swollen."

I'm glad Betty thought they were only a little swollen, because spit was coming out of the corner of her mouth, and her lips were as big as my ass. Everyone in the salon was laughing and staring at her.

Betty said, "Lucy, I need a babysitter. I promised to watch my granddaughter next week, but I'm having my eyebrows tattooed. Why should I change my appointment because my daughter wants to go away for the weekend? My beauty comes first." She never did babysit: she cancelled.

I walked away that day shaking my head. I was glad Betty wasn't my grandmother.

A client of ten years named Leslie, came into the salon crying.

"Lucy, can you do my hair right way? I have a problem."

"Leslie," I replied, "let me ask my next client if she'll let you go first." She did, so Leslie went to get her hair washed.

Leslie had breast cancer in 1996 and the breast was removed. She had had reconstructive surgery and was clear of cancer. I couldn't imagine what her problem could be know. Leslie was seventy-two and very rich.

While I was doing Leslie's hair, she told me she was upset because her plastic surgeon in Florida refused to give her a third facelift because he felt it wouldn't be safe.

Between you and me, Leslie had been pulled so tight from all her plastic surgeries that her toes were lifting off the ground. Leslie was on her way to New York to visit a new plastic surgeon who knew nothing about her past surgeries or previous cancer.

The reason for Leslie having this surgery was because, when she was babysitting her five-year-old great granddaughter, the child said, "Grandma, how old are you? Ninety?" Leslie called her great grandchild a spoiled brat and was convinced her granddaughter told the child to say something about Grandma's age.

Leslie had her facelift and died of recurring cancer two years later. She was warned.

Chapter Twenty-Two:
Everyone Has Someone Somewhere

I was checking my appointments for the day when I noticed Sherry was coming in for a restyle. When I met Sherry ten years ago, we made an instant connection. Neither one of us had children.

Sherry was sweet, naive and had a good personality. She was married for twenty years. Her husband George died and left her a ton of money. She hadn't dated in five years. She was a brunette and had long straight hair. I couldn't wait to give her a restyle. I'd been thinking about how to restyle Sherry's hair all day.

Sherry arrived at 1:30 and gave me a free hand to do whatever I wanted to her. I decided to cut her hair seven inches above her shoulders with bangs and a single flip on the ends. Fine blonde highlights would give her face life.

While I was cutting Sherry's hair, she said, "Lucy, I'm in love. It's five years since George died and no one has ruffled my feathers since, but I met a fellow named Juan. He is Latin, gorgeous, and forty-one. I don't think he has any money. I'm in love and money shouldn't matter, right, Lucy?"

"No, Sherry. Just give me all your money and you and Juan can be equal." Sherry chuckled and I said, "Sherry, do you know anything about him or his past? It wouldn't hurt you to be careful. How long have you been dating Juan?"

"Just one month. I met him at the country club."

"Have you met anyone in Juan's family yet?"

"No, but he's never been married or in love until he met me."

"Sherry, go slow and enjoy Juan. Don't go rushing into anything."

Lucille Fordin

"Okay, Lucy, I value your opinion. You're not just my hairdresser. You're my friend. We're going to the Bahamas for the weekend on his friend's yacht. I'll see you in two weeks." Sherry was glowing. She loved her hair, and I was proud of my work. We kissed good-bye and she made an appointment in two weeks for a hair blow. I couldn't help but think how naïve Sherry was.

Two weeks later Sherry came in to the salon and started to tell me an unbelievable story.

She had a glorious time in the Bahamas. Juan's friends were a little wild. They were drinking, doing drugs, and the girls couldn't keep their clothes on. When Juan saw that she was upset with the situation, he immediately got everyone under control. He had words with the two guys, and the girls were told to keep their clothes on. He also told them not to do drugs in front her.

At the end of the weekend Juan couldn't find his wallet. He said to Sherry, 'I must have gotten pick-pocketed. Would it be okay if we used your charge card? I'll pay you the minute we get back.'"

"Sherry, you didn't give him your charge card?"

"Yes, I did, Lucy, and the minute we got back he gave me the money. See, Lucy? There's nothing to worry about. Juan wouldn't hurt me; he loves me. He's so good-hearted. Someone he knew on the island asked him to bring a package back for his sister who lives in Florida. When we got back, Juan went directly to deliver the package to a woman.

"Sherry, what was in the package?"

"I don't know. Juan said nothing to worry about."

When she got home her house had been robbed. Thank God she gave her maid the weekend off so she was never in danger. Juan tried to convince her that maybe the maid had something to do with it, but Sherry knew better. The robbers knew exactly how to cut the wires to the alarm. Juan was sure he set the alarm himself. She had insurance on the jewelry. There was some cash missing.

I said to Sherry, "This sounds a little strange. Please be careful. Do you think after such a short time Juan should have access to your alarm system? I should say not. What about your charge card? That package could have been anything. Please be careful, Sherry."

"Lucy, Juan asked me to marry him and I said yes."

"Sherry, you should be happy."

"I was, but someone stole George's Rolls Royce out of the garage. It was the one thing George loved. The police haven't found it yet. I'm sure I'll never see it again."

"Sherry, what does Juan do for a living?"

"He's an investment broker. As soon as his investment goes through, he'll be a rich man, but he needs fifty thousand dollars by Monday or he'll lose everything. So if I lend him the money, I'll be an investor with him. Fifty thousand dollars can't hurt me. Juan will be a winner, not a loser, and in a month we'll fly to Las Vegas and get married. I can start the new year as a married woman."

"Sherry, please hire an investigator. At least see what his background is. You haven't met one member of his family yet, and I don't want to hear that he has no family. Everyone has someone somewhere."

"Lucy, there you go again, not trusting anyone."

"Yes, I know, but it seems funny that all these instances just started happening since you met Juan. Sherry, come on! You mean to tell me none of this seems strange to you? Sherry, I'm sorry I sound so negative. I don't mean to, but I've seen a lot of nice women get taken for a lot of money in this salon. If you're happy, I'm happy for you. Please be aware and be careful."

A couple of weeks went by and Sherry came into the salon. She was very depressed. She was squirming around in the chair and I had to tell her to sit still so I didn't burn her. She looked up at me and said, "I should have listened to you, Lucy." Then she broke down in tears.

"Sherry, calm down and tell me what happened. Maybe I can help you."

"It's too late for help now. Juan told me the investment went sour and we lost our money. Then someone charged a hundred thousand dollars on my charge card. The police said I was conned. I didn't believe them so I hired an investigator like you said. Juan disappeared. His apartment was empty. I found out that the yacht wasn't his friend's; it was stolen."

"Sherry, they probably brought drugs back in the package he delivered."

Lucille Fordin

"The woman has disappeared also. All seven of them worked together. The FBI has been trying to catch them for a while now, but they kept getting away. Oh, how could I have been so stupid?"

"Sherry, I'm convinced that one day they'll get what's coming to them. At least you are still alive and, well, that's all that counts. Women with your kind of money have to be careful nowadays. So please, in the future, don't be afraid to have your men checked out. Five hundred dollars to a PI could have saved you 150 grand, George's Rolls Royce, and all this grief from the very beginning. You haven't been raised in the streets like I have, and believe you me, there are more creeps out there than you can imagine. Look at how happy Jonathan and I are. But I went through my share of creeps, and so have a lot of other people. Get some professional help if you need to, or take a trip to Europe. Maybe that will make you feel better."

Sherry thanked me for listening to her and for not saying 'I told you so' . . . at least not in so many words.

Con men come in all shapes and sizes. Anybody who thinks that they're safe up against one of them has a lot to learn. Some swindlers are so smooth, you don't even know you're being taken until it's way too late. The money doesn't mean anything to a person that's rich. It's peanuts to them. But you never forget the pain of being stupid enough to get taken in by one of those rip-off artists.

Women are not the only ones who get ripped off. Men are just as vulnerable when they're in love. Take Jessie, a client of mine.

Jessie was fifty-two, short and chubby. He was raised on a farm in Georgia. His father worked like a dog, and when Jessie's mother ended up in a wheelchair from multiple sclerosis, he gave up his life to help take care of the farm and his mother. He never married. When Jessie's mother passed away, his father was eighty-four and never truly recovered from his wife's death.

A month before his father's death, he told Jessie that he saw his mother dancing at the bottom of his bed.

The following week his father died in his sleep with a big smile on his face.

Jessie sold the farm in Georgia and moved to Florida, and that's when he met Patty. Patty was forty-five, short, with dark hair, not too attractive, but very sweet. Patty was standing in front of a restaurant looking in her purse when Jessie pulled up to the valet and started toward the door. Patty bumped into him and dropped her purse. Jessie bent down to help her pick up everything. Patty told him her date didn't show up and she had no way home. Jessie invited her to dinner. That was his first mistake. She accepted, naturally.

Three weeks later Jessie came in and brought Patty. They were going to a party. When they left I noticed my favorite brush for blow-drying hair was gone.

When Jessie came in three weeks later, I decided to push the conversation. "Jessie, I'm so glad Mr. Davis sent you to me when you moved to Florida last year. They're very good clients and nice people, and I can see that you are a very nice man. How's that sweet girlfriend of yours? Did you enjoy the party you went to?"

"Yes, Lucy, what a great party! I made a lot of new friends. Patty is so outgoing. We knew everyone by the end of the evening, but a strange thing happened. Mrs. Davis found her bedroom door opened. The next day she discovered two of her rings were missing. I had the same thing happen to me. My watch disappeared. Lucy, Patty needs a haircut. When can I bring her in?"

"Is Saturday good, Jessie?"

"Yes. We'll see you then."

Saturday came, and after Patty left I noticed my scissors were missing. I decided to forget about it. Saturday afternoon Jessie called and asked Rosie if she found his wallet. He said he paid Patty's bill but when he went to get gas his wallet was gone.

In the months to come, every time Jessie came in he had another story to tell. It seemed like something was missing every time he had been with Patty. Jessie wasn't putting two and two together yet. I wanted to help him, so I decided to set a trap.

The next time Patty came in for her hair appointment, I left seven items on my station. When she left there were only six. Another pair of scissors disappeared.

The next time Jessie came in for a haircut, I decided it was time to have a little talk. I started cutting Jessie's hair. I was a little nervous, and didn't know how Jessie would react when I told him I didn't want Patty,

Lucille Fordin

the kleptomaniac, in the salon again. Just as I was ready to tell him, Jessie said, "I have to get out fast. I have a doctor's appointment. I feel like I'm losing my mind. Last week I went to the bank and after I got home I didn't remember what I did with the money. Patty convinced me that my cleaning girl stole the money. When I approached her, she started denying it and burst out crying. The Davises have had things missing also, so we both fired her."

"Oh no, Jessie, are you sure it's the cleaning girl? Um, Jessie, can I be blunt with you? I should have told you sooner, but I wasn't sure until last month when I set a trap. You're not going to like what I'm about to say."

"Lucy, what is it?"

"I've been listening to similar stories from the Davises, the Solos, the Briers, and many others. Everyone has had something missing after Patty visited their condos, including me."

"Lucy what are you insinuating?"

"Hear me out, Jessie. You're such a nice man. Someone would think you were raised on a farm," I said with a chuckle.

I wanted to just die. I put my big foot in my bigger mouth. I was only joking when I mentioned the farm. But boy, was this guy naïve!

"Lucy, Patty's family was killed in a car accident. She's an only child. The poor thing is all alone, except for me. I want to marry her."

"No," I blurted out. "Listen to me, Jessie. Think back. Patty was there every time things were missing. I noticed brushes and scissors missing after she left the salon, so I decided to set a trap because I thought I was losing my mind misplacing things, just like you. Every time Patty left, something was missing from my station. I decided to just let it go. I figured you would catch on eventually. You don't need a doctor. You need to set a trap. I think an innocent cleaning girl got blamed and punished, and Patty did it all. Jessie, I think you're in love with a kleptomaniac."

Jessie was upset and said, "Lucy, you're wrong about Patty."

"Jessie, I'm sorry if I spoke out of turn, but I'm one hundred percent sure it was her."

Jessie stormed out. I figured I'd never see him again. I certainly didn't care if I ever saw Patty darkening my salon door again.

Two months went by and I noticed Jessie had an appointment. I was a little nervous because I didn't know what to expect. Jessie was waiting for me at my station. I tip-toed over and said, "Hi, Jessie. Are you still mad at me?"

"No, Lucy. You're not going to shave my head bald are you?" We laughed. "I owe you a big, fat apology. Patty was a thief. I was in love and couldn't see past my nose. Mr. Davis was suspicious before you and had checked out Patty's past. She has a record a mile long. She took off and disappeared before we could have her arrested. I'll be careful from here on in, and heed your warnings too. The trap worked, but my heart was broken. I lived on a farm for so long I forgot what the real world was all about. Tell your husband he's a lucky man. Can we be friends again?"

"Of course, Jessie. I guess cows and pigs are pretty straightforward critters to deal with, huh? I do apologize for hurting your feelings. Give me a hug, Jessie, and I'll see you next month."

Chapter Twenty-Three:
Just One of the Girls and The Disease To Please

Trying to be one of the girls with the disease to please has caused me to not stop eating. I look like two-ton Tessie. It's diet time. I've been so happy lately that one day I woke up and was sixty pounds heavier! I guess too much happiness is a bad thing.

I was watching TV and Oprah was starting her diet too. She's really someone to look up to. That's who inspired me. I started out as she did, with a lot of pain and not a pot to piss in, so to speak. She made it on her own and so have I. She was fat and I was fat, and we both have been on every diet in creation. I thought I might have overactive fat cells. Yeah, right.

My overactive fat cells consisted of my hand going from the table to my mouth. With the help of Oprah's show, I lost seventy pounds and, together, my employees lost three hundred pounds. Thanks, Oprah. I watch her every chance that I get, but when you own a business you don't just work your forty hours and go home. You end up working sixty, seventy hours a week, and sometimes more. Dieting becomes difficult, eating became my friend.

I found out that it becomes very lonely at the top. I needed more food. Friends and family, especially men who thought I was a dodo or just plain stupid, were finding out that I was capable of making something out of my life. My hard work and perseverance led me to be a winner. I had the need to please myself this time, not others.

I did have one problem; I never thought school was very important. I only wanted to be a hairdresser. Well between the payroll, the bills, taxes, ordering supplies, and so on, I now know I should have paid a little more attention in school. I can't go anywhere without a calculator. I

Lucille Fordin

used to have a problem with trying to explain myself clearly, but I've learned how to do all that. I still am a very slow reader. I find myself reading the same line three times before I comprehend what's being said. You only have to show me once and I'll do the rest. I'm sure there are a lot of people out there who are just the same.

I feel pretty lucky now that Jonathan does all of the bookkeeping for me. But like most kids, I thought I knew it all. You never know where you're going to end up in life, so you better be prepared for the good times and the bad times to come.

I've always considered myself "one of the girls," at the salon, but one day one of my employees said to me, "Stop trying to act like you're one of us, because you're not. You own your own business. I'll never be lucky enough to have what you have."

I wanted to smack Joanne in her face, but I didn't. Joanne was a good hairdresser, but very jealous of everyone. She had a drinking problem. It started to effect her attitude at work.

One day she started an argument with a client and I fired her. She didn't belong in my family at the salon.

Joanne tried to hurt me with her remark and she did, but I didn't let her know it. On the way home that evening I started to cry. I felt so lonely. Most of the people around me-in the Country Club, in my neighborhood—were rich. I'm not really in their league, either. How could she say I was lucky? I worked day and night and I had no real girlfriends to speak of. I worked just like my employees, if not harder. I could party like them, and I treated everyone the way I wanted to be treated, but I was the boss.

For the second time that year, Oprah's show helped me. I was sitting on the bed wondering, Where do I belong? I switched on the TV and saw Oprah reading a letter from a viewer, telling her to "stop trying to act like you're one of us." I could feel her pain as she tried to explain. Her show has helped me in so many ways. It was my steppingstone into reality. I became proud of who I was.

A boss has to be a boss. I'm not just one of the girls. I'm stronger than most, and that's why I made it. I lost my need to please the whole world that day and I became a new person with a better attitude. I finally grew up with confidence.

I will never stop being a very generous and giving person. I enjoy giving to other people before I give to myself, but I learned how and where to draw the line.

Oprah's love for books gave me the courage to write this book. I could go on and on about Oprah because I think she is smart and beautiful. I bet she even has a good heart. It comes right though the TV screen. She's the only woman I ever wanted to meet just to say "I understand," and, "You know, you are just one of the girls!"

Well, Oprah helped me again. In April 2000, my husband had a mild heart attack and six months later, back surgery. For nine months I'd been taking care of him and the business all by myself. My mother-in-law was just in the hospital for three months. My father was visiting me in my house for the season. The husband of Sandy, my adopted step-mother, passed away, and I was trying to help her when a client called and wanted me to come to the hospital to do her hair. For the first time in my life I had to say, "I'm so sorry, but I can't right now." I explained why, and I thought she would understand, but she didn't. Life sometimes seems like the opera singer warming up her voice: "Me, me, me." I felt like I was losing my mind.

I was exhausted, crying, and punishing myself because I said, "No." I turned on the TV and Oprah happened to be on the Rosie O'Donnell Show. "Now that I'm over my disease to please, I'll be fine," she said. The way Oprah and Rosie were discussing this Disease to Please made perfect sense to me. I listened to what Oprah had to say about different kinds of selfishness and spreading oneself too thin. She did it again for me.

I stopped crying and had a good talk with myself regarding others' opinions and how I was no longer going to live my life according to them. They say that's something you learn after high school; some of us take longer than others I guess.

Oprah is so honest; she always made sense to me. If one sentence like "The Disease to Please" from her, caught by chance when I was watching the Rosie show, could so profoundly help me, then just imagine how many others she helped every day. Thank you, Oprah. You'll always be special to me, and I know I'm not alone.

Chapter Twenty-Four:
What Was That Noise I Heard, Larry?

    Women hairdressers experience the same sexual advances that male hairdressers experience. Our clientele is about eighty percent women. Gigi, an excellent hairdresser, is Latin and very hot-blooded, pretty, and energetic. Men just go crazy for her. Every once in a while, she accepts a date with a client.
    Larry DuSha was gorgeous. He had been a client for only a year. Larry was six feet tall, with sandy blond hair and baby blue eyes. All heads turned when he entered a room.
    Larry cames to Florida four times a year on business. He was very private about his life. He was thirty-three and had never married, which always seemed strange to me. Women threw themselves at him constantly, and with all the traveling he did, I guess he had no time for a family.
    As I walked by Gigi's station one day, I heard Larry say, "Gigi, it's just a date. Please don't say no again. I'm single and you're not dating anyone. Please have dinner with me tonight, with no strings attached. I hate to eat alone, and I really would like you to keep me company. I will not take no for an answer. What time should I pick you up?"
    The next day Gigi told us all about her date. She said she was in love. Larry was a perfect gentleman. He picked her up and took her to a beautiful Italian Restaurant on the water in Ft. Lauderdale. The owner of the restaurant didn't even give them a menu. They took care of Larry like he was the President. The food was exceptional and it never stopped coming. (If I had been there, there wouldn't have been any leftovers.) Customers were coming in and saying hello to Mr. DuSha like he was a king. He and Gigi were going out again that night, and I couldn't wait to see where he took her.

Lucille Fordin

The next day, Gigi told me he picked her up that evening and they had dinner on a yacht. He gave her a dozen yellow roses.

On the yacht, over dinner, Larry said, 'Gigi, I do a lot of business with the client who owns this yacht. When I'm in Florida, I have access to the yacht any time I want it."

Gigi asked Larry, "What kind of business do you do?"

"Let's not talk business. Someone as beautiful as you shouldn't have to worry about such things. You should be waited on hand and foot every day of your life. Gigi, I can give you the life you deserve." That should have been Gigi's first clue that something was not kosher.

The servants served dinner and Gigi got the white glove treatment. She and Larry lay under the stars and talked for hours. She went home wondering, Why didn't he try to sleep with me? Men are usually all over me, but this one . . . well maybe he's just trying to be conscientious.

"Lucy," Gigi said, "I can't wait to see Larry again. I'm not sure if he really likes me."

"Why do you say that, Gigi?"

"Well, he didn't try to sleep with me, and I admit I wanted him to very badly. I didn't think I should make an advance. I don't want him to think I'm a whore. What should I do?"

Just then a delivery came for Gigi — beautiful red roses thanking her for a beautiful evening. Every day that week a different colored dozen roses came to the salon, and the place was starting to look like a funeral home.

The following week Larry came in and told Gigi he had to fly out of town on business and would be back in a month.

Like clockwork, a month later Larry came straight to the salon from the airport. Larry said, "Lucy, can I speak to Gigi for a second?"

"Yes Larry, but she has to finish her client. She'll be done in five minutes. Mr. Danta is in a hurry." Larry looked impatient and pissed off. Fifteen minutes later Gigi came out and walked up to Larry and kissed him. She was so excited.

Larry blurted out, "Gigi, don't you think you took a long time cutting that man's hair? I didn't like the way he was looking at you."

"Larry, don't be jealous. He's just a client" Gigi asked me if she could trim Larry's hair for free.

I said, "Yes."

While she was cutting Larry's hair I could hear them arguing. As he left the salon, he said, "I'll pick you up after work, Gigi. Be ready at six." Then he stormed out the door.

The following week Larry was around constantly. He'd drive Gigi to work, pick her up for lunch, and then bring her back. Then he would return and pick her up at the end of the day.

I didn't like what I was seeing, but had to mind my own business, until one day Gigi came in crying.

"Lucy, can I talk to you? I'm so confused. Larry is so jealous that he goes crazy if someone looks at me. He actually asked me to marry him. I told him, no, it was too soon. I don't know anything about his life or his business. Everywhere we go, people are waiting on him hand and foot, and last night something strange happened after dinner. While we were having dessert, the owner of the restaurant said to Larry, 'Can I speak to you alone?' While Larry was in his office, a man who was sitting alone having dinner approached me.

"'You're too beautiful to be left sitting here alone,' he said. I could tell he was little high. As he put his hand on my arm I tried to tell him I wasn't interested. Larry came up behind the man, grabbed his arm and almost broke it off.

"Larry was in a rage. 'Don't you ever touch my woman,'" he said. "'I better never see your face in this restaurant again or you'll be fucking sorry.'"

Larry told her it was her fault for flirting with the guy. "Lucy, I wasn't flirting. We went back to his luxury hotel and made love all night. It was like nothing ever happened."

Larry showed up the next day to take Gigi out to lunch. When she returned, she was a little angry. Her one o'clock appointment came in early and went to Renaldo because he couldn't wait.

Larry sized up the situation and in a disgusted voice said, "Gigi, quit your job and move in with me. I'll take care of you. Let's go now."

"No," Gigi said. "Lucy is my friend and I like my job. I told you I had to be back by twelve thirty."

Larry was enraged and everyone knew it. He stormed out of the salon. Gigi was upset all afternoon and took it out on her clients. When

Lucille Fordin

Larry walked in at six to get Gigi, he didn't say hello to anyone. He just said to Gigi, "Let's go!"

The next day Gigi was wearing a five-carat engagement ring.

For the next six months Larry was coming in and out of town and still didn't move to Florida. I just knew something wasn't right.

One evening Gigi and Larry went to his client's house for dinner. Larry had a suitcase with him. They were leaving and Gigi was in the car when Larry said, "I'll be back in a minute. I forgot something."

He left and was gone for a few minutes. All of a sudden Gigi heard a loud bang. It sounded like a gunshot. Larry came out, put the suitcase in the car and drove away.

Gigi asked Larry what the noise was, but he told her to mind her own business.

Gigi came to work the next day and said, "I'm breaking up with Larry tonight."

A couple of hours later Larry came to the salon and told Gigi he had to leave town for a while and wanted her to go with him. She refused and tried to give him the ring back, but he wouldn't take it. He started cursing at her and then grabbed her by the arm. I threatened to call the police if he didn't leave. Everyone in the salon was scared. Finally, he just left, thank God. Flowers came every day for the next week and then they stopped. No phone calls and no more flowers.

A couple of weeks later Gigi got a call from Larry; he was in jail, accused of murder.

I told Gigi, "Gigi, it's time to walk away. Sell the ring and send him the money. You were giving it back anyway. Don't get involved otherwise."

Gigi told me I was right, and she would never date another client.

One day we were told Larry was convicted of murder. The prison guards soon found Larry DuSha dead in his cell.

Life can be awfully scary. We never know who's coming into and out of the state of Florida, with its huge seacoast and multicultural population.

Chapter Twenty-Five:
Now Who Would Buy Somebody a Car On a Maybe?

I went to Publix to get a stick of pepperoni, cheese and bread. The salon was busy and my employees needed a pick-me-up. When I returned, I caught the shrimp, Pepe peeking through the corner window of the salon. In a loud, angry voice, I said, "Pepe, you were told to stay away from me and the salon. No more games."

Everyone inside the salon was looking out at us while we were screaming at each other. I was eye to eye with the shrimp. All I could smell was garlic on his breath. It was gross. I felt like throwing up in his face. He called me everything from a bimbo to a bitch.

I called him a jerk, a smelly little squirt, a male chauvinist pig and a loser.

He wouldn't quit screaming, so I ran into the salon and grabbed the can of horse manure that I had saved for this special moment. I ran back outside and threw it in his face. All I could hear were people cheering and laughing. Little Pepe was really pissed off. He stunk like Pepe Lepew, the skunk from the cartoons.

After the shock wore off, Pepe grabbed a handful of the horse manure from his face and threw it at me. I ducked so fast that it missed me and hit someone behind me. That's when I noticed the crowd of people standing behind me. They were cheering me on, and people in the salon were laughing. It was another Candid Camera moment. From the corner I could see the security cops coming. All of sudden, Pepe raised

Lucille Fordin

his baby finger and forefinger, pointing and screaming at me, trying to put the evil eye on me.

I grabbed my stick of pepperoni out of the bag which I dropped on the ground and hit him across the hand. I broke that evil eye real fast.

As Pepe turned and started to run, he said, "You'll never get rid of me, you bimbo." The security cop grabbed him and asked me if I wanted to press charges.

I put a restraining order on him. He was out of business three months later. I had won the war!

The salon was very busy. There was not a seat left in the waiting area, and I was running back and forth like a maniac. The maid called off sick. It was only eleven o'clock, and I was already exhausted. I got the broom to sweep up the hair from haircuts when a woman tripped over her own foot and spilled her coffee. I wiped the coffee off the floor. Just then a very talented hairdresser named Michele started throwing a fit because his client was ten minutes late. Michele had worked for me for seven years. I ran to his station to calm him down. Thank God, he calmed down fast. I was in no mood for petty attitudes. I did my client and started doing laundry. Towels were everywhere. (One thing I'm known for is keeping the salon immaculate.) This craziness went on all day. Twelve hours felt like fifty.

Mrs. Long had been going to Michele for nine years. She was a dear, sweet woman. She was in a car accident when she was thirty years old and never drove again. Mr. Long, a very wealthy man, by the way, always drove his wife to the salon. Periodically, when Michele ran late with one of his clients, I would sit and talk to Mr. Long.

Mr. Long told me to quit cleaning and come sit with him. Within five minutes, Mr. Long asked me out on a date. I was shocked. I never thought this man cheated.

I said to Mr. Long, "I'm flattered. You're a very nice guy, but I could never hurt your wife. You're a married man and I'm a married woman. Here comes your wife. She's beautiful. See you next week." I took off like a bat out of hell.

Mr. Long was very persistent. The following Thursday when he came in with his wife, he said, "Lucy, come talk to me."

"Mr. Long, I'll be there in a minute. I have to finish ordering my products." I tried to stay as busy as possible, but Mrs. Long still wasn't ready. I felt forced to talk to him. I tried everything I could to keep his mind off me. "I heard your children are coming down for the holidays, Mr. Long."

"Forget my children. Go out with me. I'm crazy for you, and I can take care of you."

"Mr. Long, you're such a kidder. You've been married for fifty years. Why would you want to cause unnecessary trouble in your life?"

"My wife hates sex and she won't let me touch her. It's her fault I've cheated on her the last twenty-five years. Can you blame me?"

I was in shock again. I thought this had been a marriage made in heaven. Mrs. Long was ready! Just in time to save me, but she didn't know it.

She thanked me for keeping George busy. She said, "He just loves talking to you. His barber retired and I want you to cut his hair now."

"Mrs. Long, that's nice, but Renaldo is the expert with men. I'll make sure he takes good care of George." No way was I cutting this man's hair.

George put his arm around my waist and said, "When Renaldo is done taking care of me, can I take care of you, Lucy?"

I pulled away from George and hoped Mrs. Long couldn't tell how uncomfortable I was. "George you're such a kidder," I said.

Mrs. Long said, "Lucy, he's always flirting. Don't pay any attention to him. He's harmless. I'll see you next week. George, let's go home. Lucy has to go back to work. She's very busy."

In the weeks to come, George would come in one day for a haircut, another day for a manicure, and a third to bring his wife. One morning George dropped off his wife and introduced me to his son and his golfing buddy.

Mr. Long said, "Honey, can we take Lucy to breakfast with us?"

"Sure, George. Lucy, do you have time?"

"Thanks, guys, I'd love to have breakfast with three handsome fellows, but I'm too busy. Thanks for asking. Maybe next time."

As I walked away, the men were smiling, whispering, and looking at me like I was their breakfast. It made me very uncomfortable. I felt like a whore and I didn't even do anything wrong. All I could think about was

Lucille Fordin

poor Mrs. Long, who knew nothing about what was going on. It made me feel ashamed.

They came back to pick Mrs. Long up and told Rosie to take her off the books for next week because Mr. And Mrs. Long were taking a trip to Las Vegas.

Mr. Long said, "Lucy, why don't you come to Las Vegas with us? We'll pay for everything."

"Thanks, but I can't."

"I heard one of the hotels are giving away a Rolls Royce."

"You can bring it home for me. I always wanted a Rolls. Have fun and win lots of money."

When George came back, he said to me, "I didn't win you the car, but if you go out with me I'll buy you one."

"Okay, George. When I see a Rolls Royce in my name out back, I'll go out with you."

Over the next five weeks, every time George came in he'd smile and say, "The car is coming." I would laugh and say, "Sure, George."

One day Rosie got a call from Mrs. Long. "Please squeeze me in for my hair. My husband died of a heart attack and I want to look good at the funeral."

We hear this statement a lot. I could never understand how widows' hair could be so important at such a traumatic time. They should have been grieving, not primping.

There was a lot of talk at the salon that week about George Long and his affairs. Mrs. Long stayed with George for the money. She caught him cheating with her best friend twenty-five years ago and on that day quit sleeping with him.

It's funny how, after people die, they become saints. We have a way of burying the past and all the bad that happens along the way.

Week after week, Mrs. Long cried and carried on and never stopped talking about Saint George. The following week, Mrs. Long's son came to the salon with his mother. While she was having her hair done, I told him how sorry I was his father had passed away.

His son, Fred, said, "Lucy, actually you're the reason I came with Mom. My father told me all about you."

"Well, there's nothing to tell, Fred. I wasn't involved with your father. He kidded around a lot but I never had an affair with him."

"Lucy, I have something to show you. Dad ordered a Rolls Royce and put your name on it. I thought you knew about it. Look at these papers. Mom doesn't know about this at all and I never want her to find out. She's been hurt enough throughout her life."

"Fred, I can't believe George ordered this car! I mean, it was a joke. When he'd make a pass at me I'd laugh and say, 'When I see a Rolls Royce pull up at the salon for me, I'll go to lunch with you.' Who'd ever think anyone on this earth would buy someone a car on a maybe? Honestly! Rip up those papers and cancel that car. I love your mother. I've known her a long time. I'd die if she ever thought I was trying to steal her husband. It was only in his head; please believe me. Let this be our little secret. Don't ever let your mother find out.

Fred hugged me and thanked me for keeping his father's secret. I've never joked around about a present again. What would I have done if George had shown up with the Rolls?

For the next five years all I heard every week from Mrs. Long was, "George was such a good husband, and he thought you were a great woman, Lucy."

Chapter Twenty-Six:
Sometimes People Make Mistakes, Otherwise Known as The Beth Principle

It was Friday morning, and I was blowing Mrs. Sholtz's hair. A client for two years, she said, "Lucy, you have to do me a favor. My daughter Beth is flying in from California and I need you to fit her in with me next week."

"Absolutely, Mrs. Scholtz. I didn't know you had a daughter."

"I haven't seen her or talked to her in two years. We're as different as day and night. Beth has finally begun returning my calls. I'm excited, but also scared that something will go wrong again."

Mrs. Scholtz didn't volunteer any more information, so I said nothing. I gave her an appointment for Beth and off she went.

Suddenly, I heard a scream from the back of the salon. I froze for a moment, and so did everyone else. I dropped my hair blower and ran like a maniac. As I got closer to the ladies room, the screams got louder. It sounded like someone was being murdered.

I tried opening the bathroom door, but it was locked. The person screamed again, although I couldn't see a light on underneath the door. I turned and noticed the whole salon was moving a little closer toward me. Within seconds, I was pounding on the door and yelling, "Who's in there? Are you okay? What's the matter? Should I call 911?" Still no answer. I could hear crying from beyond the door. I asked the employees if anyone knew who was in the ladies room. The answer was "No." Just then I heard a voice say, "Lucy, get me out of here! I'm scared!" I realized it was Mrs. Mosk.

Lucille Fordin

"Mrs. Mosk, should I break down the door? Is the lock broken?" Mrs. Mosk said, "I don't know. The lights went out and I'm afraid to move."

I finally convinced her to unlock the door. I told her that the bathroom light had burned out. Mrs. Mosk was crying and standing in a puddle of pee. I grabbed some towels and a dye apron and went into the ladies room with a flashlight to get Mrs. Mosk cleaned up. She kept saying, "I'm sorry, Lucy, I'm afraid of the dark."

I calmed Mrs. Mosk down by telling her it would be our secret that she wet her pants. I would tell everyone that she spilled her coffee when the lights went out. As I pulled her pants off, I realized I was face to face with a wet, bushy vulva. I felt as if I were in the rain forest. Yuck! I put her pants in the washing machine and grabbed the stepladder to change the lights in the ceiling.

By the time I was finished being the maintenance woman, Mrs. Mosk was telling her story to the employees and clients and everyone was laughing.

The following week Mrs. Scholtz came in with Beth. Things seemed to be going well and I was happy for them. Beth asked me if I was married. I said, "Yes."

She said, "I don't know anyone in Florida, I need a friend to have dinner with. Will you have dinner with me, Lucy?"

We seemed to be hitting it off, so I said, "Sure, I'll have dinner with you." Beth was 5ft. tall with dark brown hair. She was very sweet, very cute, and around thirty years old.

The following week Mrs. Scholtz came in a day early to get her hair done, and I said, "How are things with you and your daughter?"

Mrs. Scholtz was very nervous. She said, "She'll be in tomorrow, Lucy. Beth told me you're having dinner with her over the weekend, that your husband will be away. Lucy, she was supposed to leave today, but decided to stay another week. I thought she was staying for me until she told me about having dinner with you.

"Lucy, I think you should cancel dinner with Beth. My daughter likes you a lot."

"Let me get this straight, Mrs. Scholtz. Your daughter likes me as a friend. She just wanted someone different to go out with her."

"You don't understand, Lucy. My daughter is gay."

"Mrs. Scholtz, in my business you come across all kinds of people. To me people are people, gay or straight or bi or whatever. It's not my place to say what anyone's sexual preference should be. As long as they treat me as a person and respect my views, then I don't have a problem with it. I'm nice to everybody."

All I kept thinking was, *Did I do something to encourage this?* But I couldn't think of anything. I thanked Mrs. Scholtz for worrying about me and I told her a lie. My husband cancelled his trip and I couldn't go out to dinner with Beth. Mrs. Scholtz was relieved; I didn't want to lose her as a client by going out with her daughter.

Beth was a nice girl, and I didn't care if she was gay. But Mrs. Scholtz made me feel so uncomfortable that I knew I had to cancel.

The following day Beth came to the salon for a haircut and blow. I noticed Beth staring at me the whole time she sat in the waiting area. I told Beth to get her hair washed and I would meet her at my station.

I asked Beth how she wanted her hair cut. The conversation went like this. "Lucy, cut my hair like yours. You have beautiful hair. Can I touch it?"

I didn't find this unusual. People are always touching my hair. I have thick hair with two shades of blonde highlights glowing through my natural (Ha! Ha!) golden brown hair.

I said, "Yes." Big mistake. Beth stroked my hair like I was her lover. I didn't know what to do, so I said, "Beth, let me cut your hair now. I'm running late."

I shut up and started cutting as fast as I could. Then Beth said, "Lucy, you have such big, pretty hazel eyes. Are your long eyelashes fake or real?"

"Thanks for the compliment, Beth. They're real. I've been blessed with a lot of hair."

Beth was very confident in herself and knew what she wanted. "Lucy, are you hairy all over?" I didn't answer her. "I love hairy women. Have you ever fantasized about being with a woman?"

Without hesitation, I said, "No, Beth, I'm happily married. Tell me about your vacation in Florida."

I kept trying to change the subject, but Beth was very persistent. Beth was squirming around in her chair, and kept brushing against my body. If

Lucille Fordin

I was on her left, she leaned to the left; if I was on her right, she leaned to the right. I was blowing her hair as fast as I could when I told her to sit still so I didn't burn her.

That didn't work. Beth said, "Lucy, I love pain. Please, burn me."

"Beth, forget the burn. How about I just beat the shit out of you?"

We laughed and then Beth gave a big sigh. She sounded like she reached a climax right in my chair. "Was it as good for you as it was for me?" she asked.

I knew what she meant, and it wasn't her haircut she was talking about. I had to get her out fast. She was getting on my nerves.

I told her I had to cancel dinner. "My husband canceled his trip and we're going away for the weekend. I hope you're not too disappointed, Beth."

"In fact, Lucy, I'm very disappointed. I thought I had a new friend. Maybe when I come down next year you'll have dinner with me. It'll be on me. I'll see you next year, love." Then Beth leaned over and kissed me on the lips. Beth licked her lips, and said, "You made my trip a pleasure." I was in shock and felt violated. She looked at me like I was a piece of prime rib.

I walked away thinking, "Sure, Beth, but you're not having me for dessert!" The next week Mrs. Scholtz canceled her appointment, and, guess what? I never saw hide nor hair of her again. The poor woman was from the old school. I felt she was so embarrassed to find out what her daughter's plans were for me that she couldn't face me.

We have plenty of gay clientele, but for me that was my first "encounter," and I didn't have a clue in the beginning. My take on the situation was that she was just looking for a friend.

I've never felt the need to experiment in that direction. I went home that night and made love to my husband like there was no tomorrow. He looked at me and said, "What did you eat for lunch, you hot tomato?"

I said, "I didn't eat anything, and I especially didn't eat a tomato." I started laughing and didn't stop until the tears rolled down my face. Then I explained the situation to my husband. Jonathan said, "I'd like to thank this Beth for a memorable evening," and then he smiled.

Gay or straight or bi, people are people and they're always looking for love. But sometimes people mistake innocence and kindness as a come on, what I now call the Beth Principle.

Chapter Twenty-Seven:
Like An Angel With A Smile On Her Face

Do you believe in ghosts? I've never seen one myself, but certain customers have told me at the salon, that they have seen a loved one that has passed or felt a presence, and have even seen objects being moved or appearing suddenly.

One day I was putting color on Brenda's hair: She is forty-two and has been a client for eight years. She said, "Lucy, I feel like I'm going crazy. One night this week I cried myself to sleep. My husband is acting very strange. I think he's having an affair. I woke up suddenly at four in the morning and the bed was empty. A cloud of smoke was wandering around the room and suddenly my mother appeared. She's been dead ten years. We were very close. I moved in with Mom to take care of her. She was dying of cancer. My husband was furious, but I didn't care.

All my Mom's spirit kept saying was, 'Don't be afraid. Leave him.' She said it three times and then she disappeared.

"When I woke up, Jerry was getting dressed for work and I confronted him. Naturally he denied everything and told me to get a job or see a psychiatrist. So I decided to go through his closet after he left. I found a phone number and I called it.

"I pretended I was Jerry's secretary and said, 'Mr. Franklin is heading out of town unexpectedly and is afraid he can't make it tonight. He's instructed me to phone and make his apologies.' Now what do you think the woman said? 'You tell Jerry I love him and I'll see him when he gets back.'

"I called Jerry at work and told him I wanted a divorce. I haven't seen him since. Lucy, have you ever seen or heard anything strange like this?" After I hesitated, Brenda asked, "Well Lucy, did you?"

Lucille Fordin

Just then the three other women getting their hair colored said, "Lucy, we're listening. Did you or didn't you?"

"Brenda, I guess I'm crazy also. In 1979, my mother died in her sleep at two in the morning on New Year's Day. My first husband was a chef, so I was alone on holidays. I would call my mom and we would talk for hours on the phone. I've always missed being with my family. New Year's Eve, all my life, at midnight, I would stop what I was doing and call home to wish Mom a Happy New Year. Dad worked a night shift, so Mom was always alone too. At twelve o'clock I called Mom,

"'Hi Lucy, Happy New Year. I love you.'

"'I love you too, Mom, and I really miss you.'

"'Lucy, listen to me. I don't feel well. I think I passed out today because when I woke up my cigarette was burned out. I only remember lighting it. When I woke up I felt like I was a teenager again. I didn't have a pain in my body and I was running up and down the stairs doing laundry and cooking for tomorrow!'"

"Brenda, Mom was very heavy and always had trouble breathing. I told Mom, 'Please go to the Emergency Room. Please call a doctor.' She refused because she didn't want to spoil New Year's for everyone. She said she'd go to the doctor's on Monday but not before.

"'Lucy, she said, "I have to wait for your brother and sister to call me. Joe's at a party and your sister is working. It's important that I don't miss their phone calls. I have to go now. I love you very much and I know you'll be okay. Take care of Roxanne and Joe.'

"I asked, 'Mom, why are you talking like this? Please don't hang up on me yet. I'm lonely.'

"She said, 'Lucy, I have to go. I must talk to your brother and sister. I love you. 'Bye.'

Mom had never hung up on me in her life. I was puzzled and started to cry. I found out later that Joe had called her right after we hung up and Roxanne called right after Joe. Brenda, Mom died right after Roxanne's phone call. She folded her hands under her face and died with a smile. When Dad got home from work, he said, "Happy New Year, honey." Mom didn't answer and he didn't want to disturb her. My brother tried to wake her up New Year's Day, but she was dead, lying there like an angel with a smile on her face.

"Mom wouldn't let herself die until she had talked to all of her children.

"A month after the funeral, I was back in Florida, home alone, sleeping. I dreamed that Mom put her hand out and said, 'Lucy I love you. I want you to come with me.'

I told Mom I loved her, but had to buy a house, have children, and start my own business. 'I must take care of Dad.' Just as my hand was ready to take her hand, my eyes opened up and I was sitting straight up on the side of the bed with my arm out in the air. When I looked at the clock, it was the same time she had died. Chills ran down my body, but I felt at peace.

"I've always been thankful that I had such a visit. I have a house and a business, but I couldn't have any children. My clients and employees are my children.

"I always wonder what would have happened if I had taken Mom's hand that night. That was the only time I ever saw her that way. I've dreamed about her two other times when I was at a low point, and each time she said, 'Lucy, don't call on me too often, honey. It's very draining on my spirit.' Then we'd talk and everything would suddenly be okay.

The women were voicing their opinions while their hair color was processing in the dye area. They had all been regular weekly clients for years. "You're all nuts. There's no life after death! Brenda's husband was right. You all need to see a psychiatrist."

"Estelle, shut your stupid mouth. I agree with both of them," June said abruptly. "I've never told anyone this, but I saw my late husband quite a few times at the bottom of my bed and I'm not crazy."

Joan jumped in and said, "My girlfriend knew her daughter was killed in a car accident before it happened. We were out having dinner and all of a sudden she got dizzy, turned white and said, 'Something is wrong with my daughter. I just got a shooting pain in my head and I saw her face! Let's go home now.' She was frantic. I kept trying to calm her down and tell her it was her imagination. We no sooner walked into her condo, when a call came from the hospital saying that her daughter had been in a serious car accident. By the time we got to the hospital, my friend's daughter was dead due to head injuries caused by the crash."

Lucille Fordin

Estelle said, "Thank God my color is done. I've heard enough of this crap. You all need to seek professional help."

Joan said, "Drop dead, Estelle. I'm glad you're leaving. Maybe you'll drown when your hair is being washed."

Rosie came running to the dye area. "What's going on, girls? We can hear you fighting all through the salon."

I told Rosie, "Everyone has a difference of opinion about seeing the dead."

Rosie looked at us like we were crazy, and said, "Seeing the dead. . . okey-dokey. Well, if you all don't keep it quiet, I'll be dead from the stress of other clients complaining about the noise. I haven't seen a good fist fight in a while. Maybe I should let you all kill each other. Then we'll see if they're ghosts." We looked at each other, then at Rosie, and we all started laughing.

I said, "Girls, it's time to break up this meeting of the minds. If I don't get you washed, the hairdressers are going to kill me, and then I'll come back and kill you."

Estelle had to have the last word. She said, "Don't tell me what to do, Queeny. I'll get washed when I'm ready."

I had enough of Estelle's arrogant mouth. "Fine. The rest of you girls get your colors washed out and Estelle can go bald. Estelle, your timer went off ten minutes ago."

Estelle jumped up fast and didn't say another word. I chuckled as I walked away. A major bad word in a hair salon is, "BALD!"

Chapter Twenty-Eight:
Keep The Tranquilizers Coming, Girls!

It was Christmas time at the salon.

When confronted with the prospect of free food, everyone's class and good taste go right down the drain. Just say, "The buffet is ready to be served," and a stampede will occur. Girls with bodies as big as my ankles become human vacuum sweepers. I'm sure you all know someone who eats like a hog when the food is free, or am I just such a good cook that no one can help him or herself?

From 8 to 10 in the morning, as people were eating everything, they kept saying with their mouths full, "It's too early to eat. Can I take a doggy bag? I'll just taste this, and this, and this, and that. I'm on a diet, so I better not eat a third plate of food.

Mr. Henderson had a manicure in the morning and a hearty breakfast. He was fifty-eight years old, widowed, and CEO of a major corporation. Around twelve he called and begged for a one o'clock appointment and got a haircut. Mr. Henderson had two large plates of food and a load of desserts. At three Mr. Henderson called and asked if he could get a pedicure at five. "Please Rosie, squeeze me in." Mr. Henderson ate so much lasagna that he looked like he was going to bust.

"Thanks," he said. "Everything was delicious" as he walked out the door.

In a joking voice I said, "I guess I won't see you for three weeks, Mr. Henderson. You have nothing left for us to do, unless you get a facial or a massage."

"Great idea, Lucy! What's for breakfast?" I had visions of him lying in bed, a victim of death by lasagna. By the way, Mr. Henderson had a massage in the morning and a facial at dinnertime. There was nothing left

Lucille Fordin

for Mr. Henderson to have done now except for a bikini wax. Thank God he didn't call the next day. I heard later that he thought he was having a heart attack, and ran to the doctor's office for tests. It must have been those last fifty meatballs he ate. The diagnosis was overeating. No heart attack.

There were mirrors everywhere in the salon, and I could see everything that happened at the buffet. There were three tables of food, and Mrs. Kendall was sitting in the corner, eating a plate of pasta and salad. She reached over, cut a piece of cake, wrapped it up in a napkin and put it in her purse. Mrs. Kendall got another plate of food, and as she was eating, she put a sandwich, a handful of candy, and some fudge balls in her purse. Mrs. Kendall felt sure no one saw her, but we all know someone always sees you.

Three other clients and I watched her the whole time. Every time Mrs. Kendall sighed in relief, thinking no one saw her and that she had got away with stealing food, the four of us became hysterical, laughing until there were tears in our eyes.

As Mrs. Kendall was paying her bill, she was having difficulty finding her wallet in her purse, so I said, "I'll help you, Mrs. Kendall." She immediately panicked and practically screamed, "Oh no, I have it." After she retrieved her wallet with great difficulty, paid and left, the ladies were still laughing. One of them said, "I'll bet she has one big fudge ball sandwich in her purse when she gets home." We talked about it for weeks.

Another woman, Mrs. Sekauley, ate five plates of food and then sat in a chair and went to sleep until her color was done. While she was sleeping, a couple of women called Rosie over and said, "I think that lady must be dead, she ate so much. Tell Rosie to check on her."

Rosie came over to me and told me what the women said and now they were all laughing. Mrs. Sekauley soon started snoring and making other strange noises. I said to everyone, "She's not dead." And then Mrs. Sekauley got real quiet and her head slowly dropped. Rosie said, "Wake her up before she gets hungry again."

Joanne said, "I think she's really dead."

Mary said, "After five dishes of food, she will probably have diarrhea all night." We all looked at each other and started laughing.

"Girls, this reminds me of the time a woman died under the hair dryer when I was working in Pittsburgh. It was terrible. She was fifty-five years old.

"I was busy that day in Pittsburgh. Two hours went by and I noticed Angie wouldn't wake up. So I gently rubbed her arm and said, 'It's time you got up.' She was like ice. We called for an ambulance, but she was already dead. They said she had an aneurysm and died in her sleep."

On that note, I felt I'd better go and check on Mrs. Sekauley. I was getting nervous. Just then Mrs. Sekauley's timer went off and she jumped up and said, "I'm hungry. I think I'll have dessert after my color gets rinsed off." Well, we all cracked up laughing like fools. Every time Mrs. Sekauley asked what was so funny, we all just laughed so hard we almost choked.

From time to time in any salon, things would disappear, like cookies, toilet paper, scissors, combs, brushes, etc. This was always a shock because we have rather wealthy people who come into the salon. This goes back to a statement you hear a lot today: "I'm entitled." I'm still trying to figure out, "entitled to what?" My mother always told me if it doesn't belong to you, leave it alone; it's not yours. You never take anything that doesn't belong to you.

A lot of businesses fold because of the "I'm Entitled Principle." My mother taught me never to rob from anyone, but there are a lot of cookie thieves out there in the world, and you all know who you are.

There were at least five hundred people in the shop that Christmas week. Clients brought their friends and families with them. Under the Christmas tree were presents for all the children and teenagers. The little kids' faces would light up with joy when they were given a present for just being in the salon at Christmas. I got more hugs and kisses from the children than I did from the adults.

On the last day of the party, the morning started out very slowly. All the employees were exhausted and I was sick of looking at food. At 8am a woman said to me, "Lucy, get out of my way. I'm starving. Can't you get the food out any faster?" She almost knocked me over to get to the egg salad. Mrs. Tomashevsky had so much food on her plate it was falling on the floor. Then she proceeded to step on it and make a holy mess. I turned to her and said, "Is this what you do at home?"

Lucille Fordin

As Mrs. Tomashevsky made a sour face at me, she turned away and spilled her coffee all over the place, but never let go of her plate. She never even apologized, and she said to me, "It's your fault. You made me nervous. Now you can clean it up."

Mrs. McLaughlin said, "You're acting like an animal. Where were you raised?"

Then Mrs. Peters jumped in and said, "How could you talk to Lucy that way after she did all this work for us? Open your mouth again and I'll get you thrown out of the club."

Just then Mrs. Tomashevsky said to Mrs. Peters, "Mind your own business, you bothersome piece of shit."

My mouth dropped open and nothing would come out. Everyone was deadly silent for a second, and then came a free-for-all attack on Mrs. Tomashevsky. I hollered, "Ladies, ladies! Stop now, please! We're all a little tired from the holidays, shopping and all, and I'm sure no one means what they're saying. Your hairdressers are ready for you; please relax, ladies. Thank you for your help."

Just then Joan pulls out a tranquilizer and gave it to me. "Lucy, here, take this pill and calm down," she said. "You're becoming excited. We're just having a little fun."

All the ladies were hysterically laughing and talking about Mrs. Tomashevsky, telling me, "This is better than being at the movies." I took the pill and half an hour later I was feeling real good.

Mrs. Tomashevsky never missed a bite. All of a sudden she said to me, "Can I take my dessert home? Those crazy women make me nervous. I can't eat so good now."

I couldn't get Mrs. Tomashevsky out of the salon fast enough. I wrapped up cake and sent her on her way. I would have given her the whole damn salon just to get her out of there.

It was a marvel that morning to watch those classy women turn into cats. It was like a street fight, although it was really just a good-natured clubhouse fight, and we laughed for weeks about it.

I announced the winners of the clients' grab bag over the intercom. Some women were cheering the winners, while the rest were complaining that they never won anything. Each bag had a beautiful set of costume jewelry (a very elegant necklace and ear-rings), as well as a brush and comb with a can of hair, spray along with a bag of candy and a rain bonnet.

Just then I announced, "You're all winners in my eyes and I love you all. Hair Network women and men are all special to me. This is my way of showing you my appreciation and, now . . . everyone take a deep breath and let's party."

I put on the Macarena tape that my nephew bought for the salon. The whole shop dropped what they were doing for a few minutes. The staff and clients were dancing like fools, laughing while each person did the dance his or her own way.

Thank God the salon mood turned around toward fun and laughter. We made it through the morning somehow, and with only six hours left before closing, I figured we had it made. Wrong again.

At 1:00pm a lady pushed a gentleman aside to get at the food. He had to hold on to the table to stop from falling. The woman's foot got caught on the leg of the table and a black forest cake went sliding. It landed on Mr. Cohen's pants and shoes.

Clients were laughing and screaming for me to come fast. Mr. Cohen screamed at Mrs. Danny. "You idiot! You're an animal!" Then they started screaming crazy things at each other.

Just then I came over. My eyes opened wide and my mouth dropped open.

I said to Mr. Cohen, "Look at all the cherries you ended up with. It's easier to eat them than it is to find them or wear them. Keep the tranquilizers coming, girls! I'm going to need all the help I can get today."

Thank God Mr. Cohen began laughing hysterically while we cleaned him up. I told him to take his clothes to the cleaners and send me the bill.

All of a sudden Mr. Cohen said, "Lucy, can I see you for a minute?"

I got so nervous my heart was pounding. I said, "I'm so sorry."

He said, "Don't be sorry. It was an accident. Mrs. Danny acted like she hadn't seen food since her Bat Mitzvah. Lucy, you did a great job and I wanted to thank you for everything. I've not had this much fun since I was a kid. I didn't know wearing a cake could be so much fun."

The rest of the day was just as crazy. I was glad it was over until next year. I sat down to catch my breath when Zane handed me a card and

Lucille Fordin

said, "Lucy, I love you. This will make you feel better." I opened the card and this is what it said:

> *"Boss. No matter how you figure it,*
> *happy employees and a pleasant work*
> *place means only one thing: Someone*
> *pretty terrific is in charge.*
>
> *Dear Lucy and Jonathan,*
>
> *I want to thank you both for always going the extra mile to make things better. I have worked for a lot of people before you, and I must say you guys are the best! I love and appreciate you more than I could ever adequately say. I love you both. Have a great year.*
>
> *Thanks again,*
>
> *Zane.*

I started to cry with joy. Just when I thought no one appreciated anything, Zane's card made me realize there would always be some people who would take everything for granted, yes, but there would also be others who appreciated what I did for them. Those were the ones who made everything worthwhile in life.

I received beautiful thank-you notes from the clients as well. One said, "Lucy I have been all over the world, and no one has ever treated us like family or given us such a party to thank us like you do."

One lady handed me the following homemade poem.

> *Dear Lucy,*
> *You know the true meaning of giving*
> *With your parties all year long.*
> *It's from your heart*
> *To do your part*
> *To make the clients*
> *Feel they belong.*
> *The coffee, bagels and cream cheese*
> *That you graciously provide each week*
> *Are a welcome treat that can't be beat,*
> *For a snack that we all seek.*
> *Your beauty shop remains on top,*
> *When it comes to being clean.*
> *The work that you do*

Comes shining through,
With your successful crew
On the scene.
You're wished the best
And I hope you're blessed
With good health
Above all of the rest.
Fill your life full of zest."
Lovingly,
Marlane

There are plenty of nice people in the world. We should always be thankful for who we are and what we have, because none of us knows what's waiting around the corner.

New Year's came in with a bang of new hope for a good new year. In the weeks to come everyone talked about the good and the bad.

Some got married, some got divorced, some found out that their children had died, some got nothing for Christmas, and some got a lot. The holidays could be very depressing for some and quite joyous for others. But life is what you make it.

Chapter Twenty-Nine:
I've Never Seen Lips As Big As My My Feet Before

I love listening to all the stories after New Year's. Some are good and some are bad. This particular Wednesday was quiet so I had time to sit with Renee in the waiting area. Michele has been doing Renee's hair for nine years and was running twenty minutes late.

Renee, a very sweet woman around forty-two years old, whose husband left her for his secretary five years earlier, met the man of her dreams. They were engaged for Christmas.

Renee said, "Lucy, how were your holidays?"

"Very good, but hectic. How were yours?"

"I got married. Look at the seven-carat diamond Jason gave me. New Year's Eve Jason told me, 'Pack your bags. I have a surprise for you.' His limo arrived at six and it took us to his private jet. As we entered the jet, there were flowers, champagne, and a violinist playing the song we danced to on our first date, the night we fell in love. I was so overwhelmed; I said to Jason, 'Where are we going?'"

Jason told Renee that he didn't want the hassle of a big wedding, and if it was okay with her, he wanted to be married in Las Vegas.

Naturally she said, 'Yes,' and off they went. They were married on New Year's Eve. The honeymoon suite had its own inside pool. The room was filled with presents and flowers. Jason gave her the engagement ring and an emerald necklace for a wedding gift. "Lucy, I'm on cloud nine! I kept thinking, 'This has to be a dream.'"

Lucille Fordin

"Renee, I'm so happy for you. Just enjoy Jason and your life. You deserve it."

Wasn't that a beautiful story? Behind every disaster there was a bright light shining for us all. It could be as unpretentious as a new coffee pot, or it could be a jet ride to Utopia.

Kerry had been coming to the salon for six years. Gigi does her hair. Kerry couldn't have children so for the last five years she had been trying to adopt a pair of twins. I walked over to Kerry while Gigi was doing her hair and said, "What did Santa Claus bring you, Kerry?" Her face lit up like a light bulb and her eyes filled up with tears.

"Kerry" I said, "I'm sorry. I didn't think that maybe something bad happened. I'm really sorry."

"No, Lucy, I'm not sad. These are tears of joy. I adopted a pair of twins, two beautiful little blond boys. They're six months old."

I was relieved that it was good news. I told Kerry that their first haircut was on the house. She was ecstatic. She finally got the Christmas present she wanted.

Patty's been coming to the salon for twelve years. Renaldo was doing Patty's hair and I was at my station, cleaning my brushes, when I heard her say, "Renaldo, would you like to have dinner with me? My divorce came through and I settled with the cheating bastard for $5 million. The key word here is, 'settled'.

I started choking and Renaldo ran to get me some water. I apologized to Patty for listening.

Patty said, "It's okay, Lucy, I have no secrets. Everyone knows that cheaten' bastard only gave me $5 million. I told everyone how cheap he is."

"Patty", I said, "that's enough money for you to live on for at least a year." I started laughing and choking again and thanked Renaldo for the water.

"Lucy, it's not funny. I was married to a cheater for twenty-five years. I should have gotten at least one million for each year. I'm pissed."

I stopped laughing real fast and continued cleaning my brushes. This woman is fifty and rich. Some of us barely get out of a marriage alive, and $5 million wasn't enough for Patty. What was wrong with this picture?

I knew Simon and Judy for seven years. This was a second marriage for both of them. One day in May while I was doing Judy's hair, she told me that she filed for a divorce, but Simon refused to let her go. Simon was a great, dear, soft-spoken man. He had been married to Judy for twenty years. Simon made his money in the stock market. He was never a well man, suffering from one health problem after another. Infections, operations, and tumors were everyday occurrences for Simon.

Simon had just found out about his kidney problem and that, without a transplant, he would die. Without any hesitation his parents, two children and sister had themselves tested. No match. He would never live long enough to take advantage of a national donors list, and so it seemed he needed a kidney immediately from a family member. Judy decided to be tested only if he agreed to give her a divorce. By a stroke of luck she was a match. Judy decided to give Simon a kidney for a Christmas present. This was a very special present from a woman who got a divorce in exchange for a kidney. She was a better woman than I. I'm not sure if I would give up a kidney to someone I hated enough to leave.

Mira had been coming to the salon for ten years. She was having a manicure with Jessie when I noticed her face was swollen like a balloon. I sat down next to Mira and said, "I hope your boyfriend Jake didn't hit you."

Jessie looked up and said, "No, Lucy, her boyfriend didn't hit her. Right, Mira? Tell Lucy what you did to your face."

"Okay, let me start at the beginning, Lucy. Jake was flying to Florida for Christmas and New Years. I haven't seen him for two months. His business keeps him traveling."

Mira was so excited. Jake had a big surprise for her for a Christmas present. She was praying for an engagement ring. So being the outlandish, self-absorbed woman that she is, she decided to get her eyes and lips tattooed for Jake for Christmas.

Two weeks before Christmas, Mira had the job done. She found she was allergic to the dye and swelled up like a balloon and blistered everywhere. She was a mess.

Jake decided to come home a few days early to surprise her. When he opened the door he almost fainted, and said, "Mira darling, are you okay? What happened to you? Who did that to you? I'll kill him."

Lucille Fordin

Mira started crying and could barely talk. She was babbling on and on. When Jake finally realized what she was saying, he started fighting with her and screaming at her.

"What the hell kind of Christmas present is this? I came here to give you an engagement ring, but I've changed my mind. You've ruined your face! Mira, I loved your natural beauty. If you would do this, what else are you capable of doing? I made arrangements for New Year's and now what am I going to do, go alone? We were going to meet big clients at the Country Club. I'm going to a hotel!" He stormed out the door.

The more Mira cried, the more her face burned from the tears. All night she packed her face in ice until her eyelashes had icicles.

She didn't hear from Jake the next day. The medication was finally working and the swelling was going down. The next morning Mira called his hotel.

She said, "Jake I'm much better now. I'll be perfect for New Year's. Please come over so we can talk. I'll never do anything like this again without discussing it with you first. We were going to get married! Please, I'm sorry. I wanted to be prettier for you Jake. Will you come over? It will be a great millennium, I promise."

"Okay, Mira", Jake said, "I'll come over Christmas Eve. I had no intentions of really working on this trip, but I started something and now I have to finish it. I shouldn't have come down early. You need two days to recuperate, and I need two days to finish my business deal. Mira honey, will your lips be normal by Christmas? I've never seen lips as big as my feet before. It was a shock. I love you and I'll make it up to you."

Mira's face shrunk back to normal. Mira and Jake made up and had a great millennium. They got engaged and planned their wedding.

Russ had a very different present for his parents. Russ has been coming to the salon since he was eighteen years old. It was a week before Christmas and Russ decided to tell his parents at Christmas time that he was gay. His parents were very old fashioned and, since he was their only child, a major shock was about to happen.

After Christmas, I asked Russ at the salon how his mother and father liked his present.

"Lucy, how do you know about the present?"

"Russ, you were talking very loud while Renaldo was cutting your hair. I was doing my client and we were both listening to your conversation. Don't be alarmed. Being honest with your parents is nothing to be ashamed of. How bad did your parents take the news?"

"Lucy, it was Christmas Eve, and I couldn't keep my secret any longer. I told Mom and Dad that I had something I wanted to tell them.

"Mom said, 'Russell, are you getting married?'

"No Mom, listen to me. You never listen to me. Don't I look different to you? I'm thirty years old and I'm tired of you two asking me when am I going to get married. The answer is never. I'm gay!"

"No one said a word for five minutes, Lucy. Then my father grabbed his chest and fell back in the chair."

"Quick, Russell, get Dad's pills on the dresser!"

"After getting two nitroglycerin pills down with a glass of water, my father just said, 'We'll talk tomorrow,' and he went to his room."

The next day wasn't easy. All day Christmas they talked. They decided that their son's sexual preference wasn't worth losing him over, but forbade him to bring a man into their home.

After New Year's, Lisa told me over a cup of coffee at the salon, that she bought her girlfriend a new Lincoln Cadillac Seville for Christmas.

Lisa was married and divorced three times. She had two children from her second marriage. Lisa lives in a beautiful, four bedroom home left to her by her third husband. Lisa was fifty-two when she had her first gay relationship. She is now fifty-five and has been in love for two years. Lisa wants to move to California and marry her soul mate.

Candy had all the employees and clients laughing for months. She's funny and wild and has been coming to Jessie for manicures for three years. Candy bought her own Christmas present: Two new vibrators. Her collection of dildos kept growing and growing. She brags about having fifteen of them. Candy said it was easier to use vibrators than go through the agony of relationships with men.

One can only wonder what a Millennium 2002 Vibrator does with its five speeds and multiple attachments.

Matt had been coming to me for seven years and he loved to gamble. Some days he was broke and some days he was throwing money around

Lucille Fordin

like it was nothing. He was a very generous guy. He told me he didn't believe in Christmas. Hum!

Matt hit the lottery with three other people and he only ended up with two million dollars. He was furious. (Now would you be furious if you ended up with two million dollars? I didn't think so.) I would order a giant pizza and eat it all by myself.

One Christmas thirty-two years ago, my parents asked me what I wanted for a gift. I said, "My own large pizza with everything on it, for me and only me." God, I remember that like it was yesterday. All my life I had to share everything with Joe and Roxanne. I wanted my own pizza, and one day I got it. I sat there and ate the whole thing myself. Boy, did I make myself sick! But it was fun. Even as an adult, look what I asked for—my own pizza. I guess that's why my butt will look like the Titanic the rest of my life.

That reminds me of the time my nephews, Matt and Jon, called me on the phone and said, "Mom is taking us out to build a snowman and we wish you were here." Boy, did that kill me because I did wish I were there all the time.

I told Matt and Jon, "When you're out there building a snowman, just make sure it has a big butt like Aunt Lucy's and then put a few dimples in it, maybe a lot of 'em. Then, instead of putting a carrot in its mouth, put a piece of pizza there instead." Boy, did we laugh.

A day later Roxanne called and said, "Are your ears ringing? We had so much fun building this Aunt Lucy snowman that we almost got frostbite trying to put the pizza in the snowman's mouth. Your nephews went to the freezer, pulled out an entire frozen pizza and shoved it in the snowman's mouth, and we never stopped laughing. We also spray-painted it.

"The next day, when we went out to take a picture to send to you, the snowman was messed up and the pizza was long gone. I guess an animal knocked over the snowman and had a real good supper. Little Matt thinks the snowman ate the pizza. We couldn't stop laughing, because no matter what we would say, he would say, 'The snowman ate the pizza!'"

Chapter Thirty:
I'm Next!

One day the salon was very busy. There was a major black-tie party at the Country Club that night. I was very excited. I had bought a very elegant gown to wear, but at that point I had to calm everyone down. Things were getting a little heated in the salon. All the hairdressers and manicurists were running late. It was just like New Year's Eve.

"I'm next."

One woman told the shampoo girl that she was next, but in the meantime she had gone to the ladies room, and when she came out, all three shampoo girls were naturally busy. What do you think she said? "I told you I was next. I'm not waiting, so get that person out of my chair."

"Jerry, you'll be next," I said, "You were in the ladies room and the shop is jammed. I couldn't wait ten minutes for you to come back while people were waiting. The shampoo girl will be ready for you in a few seconds."

Jerry screamed out loud, "I don't wait for anyone! I told you I was next!"

You'll never believe what Jerry did next. She sat down right on top of the woman who was in the shampoo chair having her hair washed.

"Help!" screamed the woman. "Someone get this elephant off me." The clients and employees started laughing hysterically. I heard another woman yell out, "It's show time!"

Well, you know, I was dumb founded. That was a first for me. Here we have a very rich woman, thinking she should always be first, actually sit on top of a strange woman's lap.

I proceeded to calm Jerry down while the other woman was screaming, "Get off of me, you bitch!" Suddenly, there was dead silence in the

Lucille Fordin

salon. Everyone's mouth was wide open and people were in shock. I pulled Jerry off the woman and sat her in a chair, gave her some water and told her to take a tranquilizer.

"Lucy, I'm so sorry. I don't know what happened to me. I'm so upset. My dress wasn't ready at the cleaners, and I had to have it let out because I gained twenty pounds. My husband doesn't feel well, so I won't know until the last minute if I'm even going to the party or not. I'm so sorry. Do you want me to leave?"

"No, Jerry, let's get your hair washed so you're ready for Pierre. He's waiting for you, and if you think you're crazy, wait until you see Pierre flip out if I don't get you ready on time. One of his clients got in Renaldo's chair earlier and he's upset."

Just then a gentleman named Frankie jumped out of Roberto's chair yelling, "What's the friggin' matter with you, Roberto? You know I never cut my eyebrows before I go to Las Vegas. It's bad luck. I'll kill you. How could you forget? You've been cutting my hair for eight years now."

Roberto started apologizing to Frankie.

"I thought you were going to the party. I'm sorry."

"Well, I'm not, and you have probably just cost me thousands."

I ran over to Frankie and said, "I'm sorry, Frankie; the haircut is on me."

"Lucy, you're lucky I don't sue you. Don't you have any control over your hairdressers? This place better hope I don't lose all my money."

"Frankie, is that a threat? I think you should leave now. You're making a fool out of yourself."

Frankie stormed out the door. This was another first for me. I never heard that cutting your eyebrows was bad luck for gamblers.

Two weeks later Frankie sent an apology to the salon along with lunch for all twenty-five employees. Thank God Frankie won two hundred and fifty thousand dollars in Las Vegas. Now he insists on having his eyebrows trimmed before every Vegas trip, claiming, "It's very good luck, you know."

All of a sudden I heard Chichi say to her client, "How do you want your hair done, Clorese? Since I feel wild, I guess I'll make your hair wild."

"Chichi, don't experiment today. I'm going to the party and I want my hair casual. What is wrong with you today? Are you crazy? Why are you so upset, Chichi?"

"Oh Clorese, my boyfriend is so jealous he's driving me crazy. And look over there. Yolanda is in Renaldo's chair. I'm so mad. I've been doing her hair for fifteen years and because of the party, she went to Renaldo."

Just then Clorese looked in the mirror and screamed at Chichi. "You ruined my hair! No wonder Yolanda went to Renaldo. You're crazy today."

Clorese screamed for me to come fast. As I approached all Chichi said was, "Oh my God, stay calm Clorese. I'll redo your hair."

"Chichi, it's time for you to take a break" I said. Please go calm down and let me redo Clorese's hair." Just to ease some of the tension, I added, "Please give Chichi a tranquilizer." Ten women yelled out at the same time, waving their hands in the air saying, "I have one." We all looked at each other and started laughing.

The day never got any better really, but we made the best of it. As we were leaving, Renaldo, said to me, "My scissors are missing. If they turn up, please put them in my drawer." As I was locking all the doors, everyone was saying goodnight.

As I started walking toward the car, I heard someone pounding on the windows, screaming, "Let me out of here, help! Lucy, open the door and let me out of here."

"Mrs. Shapiro, where were you when we were saying goodnight and locking up?"

"I was in the dressing room getting dressed. I got dizzy, so I sat on the chair and closed my eyes. When I came out, no one was here. What's even worse is I almost missed the party. What if you didn't hear me? What would I have done?"

"Mrs. Shapiro, security would have called me. All you had to do is unlock the door from the inside and the alarms would have gone off."

Just then a few employees hollered, "Is everything all right?" I told them what had happened and we all started laughing and couldn't stop.

The party was a success. What an elegant affair for elegant people! There were some people who started from scratch, along with people who were born into rich families. I couldn't help thinking how calm and sweet everyone was. I guess you wouldn't believe these were the same women and men screaming all day in the salon.

All through the following week, everyone was talking about what a good time he or she had and how beautiful everybody's hair looked. Oh, and the gossip, gossip, gossip.

"Yolanda looked like she was trying to screw every man she got near."

"Did you see how fat Jerry got? I heard at the salon she had to let her dress out. She looked like Miss Hippo Hips."

"Didn't Lynn have three facelifts? If they pull her face any tighter she'll explode."

"Just how old is Frankie's Las Vegas girlfriend?"

"She's sixteen. He was supposed to go to Vegas and miss the party. He went crazy because his eyebrows got trimmed, so he didn't leave until this morning."

"What about Alma flirting with Joanne's husband? It looks as if Alma could be his fourth wife. I'm sure leaving her husband is no problem. I heard he is cheating with his secretary. Just think, Joanne could get a new stud and at least fifteen million dollars. How could she go wrong?"

"Gino's lucky he sent his bodyguards and didn't show up. I heard he's involved in some shady business."

"How about Amber? What a fool. Are you sure that wasn't her son she was with? It looked as if she was burping him all night."

"Burping? You must be kidding! She had his face buried in her boobs all night. She always said when you're rich you have the option to buy a new or used car. 'I chose a hot Lamborghini.'"

Just then I stepped in and said, "Ladies, aren't we being a little catty, are we?"

"No , Lucy, we're not."

"This is more fun than being at the party."

"How was your evening, Lucy?"

"You better be careful or someone will snatch your Jonathan from you."

"Well, girls, it's nice to see we're all back to normal." As I walked away I heard someone say, "Jonathan is hot stuff. I'm prettier and thinner than Lucy; he should be with me. I'm going to give him a climax he'll never forget."

Some people measure love by how much money a person has, some by how you look, some by education, some by personality, and so on. But when you feel those tingles in your body, you know you have the right one.

Chapter Thirty-One:
You Don't Have To Be A Genius

Writing a book like this was always my mother's dream. She never lived long enough to fulfill her dreams. I would never have written it if it weren't for her drilling into my head, "You can do anything you want to do if you want it badly enough. The whole world is open to you and anyone who wants to be a winner. Never say you can't do it." I would not be where I am today if her love didn't stay with me forever. I know one day I'll see her again. I just want to tell her thanks and how much I love her.

Life can be a happy journey or a lonely journey. It's your choice. The only way to make your dreams come true is to make them come true. Believe in yourself and you will succeed.

One day I hope to see all of you visit Hair Network. Bring in a copy of this book and I'll sign it for you. But that's not necessary either; just come on down. I promise you'll have a pleasant experience.

I thank all my women who helped me through my life and taught me not to be afraid of rich people. Through all my experiences, I have found out you don't have to be a genius to make it in life. Hard work and determination can usually get you wherever you want to go. So if people ever tell you that you're stupid, get them back by making something out of yourself.